The
Full-Body
Fat
Fix

The Full-Body Fat Fix

**The Science-Based 7-Day Plan
to Cool Inflammation, Heal Your Gut,
and Build a Healthier, Leaner You!**

Stephen Perrine

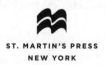

ST. MARTIN'S PRESS
NEW YORK

The information in this book is not intended to replace the advice of the reader's own physician or other medical professional. Before undertaking any of the diet or exercise recommendations provided in this book, you should consult with a qualified doctor or professional health provider. The author and the publisher do not accept responsibility for any adverse effects individuals may claim to experience, whether directly or indirectly, from the information contained in this book.

First published in the United States by St. Martin's Press, an imprint of St. Martin's Publishing Group

www.stmartins.com

Designed by Meryl Sussman Levavi

Library of Congress Cataloging-in-Publication Data

Names: Perrine, Stephen, author.
Title: The full-body fat fix : the science-based 7-day plan
    to cool inflammation, heal your gut, and build a
    healthier, leaner you / Stephen Perrine.
Description: First edition. | New York : St. Martin's Press,
    2024. | Includes bibliographical references and index.
Identifiers: LCCN 2023058065 | ISBN 9781250289520
    (hardcover) | ISBN 9781250289537 (ebook)
Subjects: LCSH: Reducing diets—Popular works |
    Inflammation—Diet therapy—Popular works. |
    Nutrition—Popular works. | Health—Popular works.
Classification: LCC RM222.2 .P43464 2024 |
    DDC 613.2/5—dc23/eng/20240118
LC record available at https://lccn.loc.gov/2023058065

Our books may be purchased in bulk for promotional, educational, or business use. Please contact your local bookseller or the Macmillan Corporate and Premium Sales Department at 1-800-221-7945, extension 5442, or by email at MacmillanSpecialMarkets@macmillan.com.

First Edition: 2024

10 9 8 7 6 5 4 3 2 1

For Dom & Henry and Anaïs & Greg

Contents

FOREWORD

Hey there, I see you.

Actually, I can see *inside* of you.

It's one of the things I love about gastroenterology: Unlike most specialists, I get to look inside the bodies of my patients. Procedures like endoscopy and colonoscopy mean that a gastroenterologist like me can get right in there, diagnose the issue, and get to work, all without needing a scalpel. It's some of the most efficient and immediately rewarding work a doctor can do.

But over the past decade, my chosen field has changed, and the work we do has become even more profound. In many ways, the medical community has finally come around to finding the gut as complex and compelling as I do. And the heart of that scientific awakening is in the microbiome.

When I was first studying medicine at NYU in the 1990s, we were taught that the microbiome—the teeming trillions of bacteria and other microbes that reside in our intestines—is responsible for just one main task: digestion. This complex ecosystem of belly bugs basically hung around in the gut and helped us process the fiber and absorb the nutrients that passed through. But beyond that, modern medicine really didn't give the microbiome a second thought.

Today, we've learned that the microbiome is, in many ways, the epicenter of our physical and emotional health. How healthy your microbiome is can have far-reaching effects throughout your body, impacting everything from immunity to blood sugar control, from our metabolism to our weight. Scientists now think of the gut as the "second brain," as we continue to learn more and more about how the microbiome helps control our hormones, our emotions, and even our energy levels. (And maybe it ought to be considered our "first brain." After all, the microbiome in our gut weighs roughly four to five pounds. The brain in our skull weighs only three!)

More than 2,500 years ago, Hippocrates, the father of modern medicine, issued an edict: "All disease begins in the gut." Today we know just how true his words were. Obesity, diabetes, heart disease, depression—even diseases of aging such as osteoporosis, sarcopenia (age-related muscle loss), and Alzheimer's disease—all have connections to the gut, a scientific fact that the world of medicine is only now relearning.

And that means that we have more power over our own health and wellness than we once thought. About 85 percent of the microbes in our guts have been shown to be beneficial; they help manufacture hormones like serotonin, the very compound that antidepressants look to boost; they help create a barrier in the lining of your intestines, protecting you against inflammatory compounds and unhealthy bacteria that cause a host of diseases; they even help regulate the immune system, impacting our ability to respond to infectious diseases from the common cold to COVID-19.

But as with any diverse population, there are some bad actors in there. When you take care of your microbiome, the beneficial microbes that aid in digestion, reduce inflammation, and protect against disease are all able to blossom. But when you're not taking care of your gut, the troublemakers start to take over. Like a handful of drunk hecklers at a comedy club, they ruin the party for everybody else—sending out inflammatory compounds, disrupting the lining of the intestines, messing with our hormones, and signaling the immune system to react in unhealthy ways.

Your microbiome is never static—it's always changing. How well you sleep, how much stress you're under, the medications you take, the exercises you do (or don't do)—they all affect the microbiome, in ways that we're still learning about. But the most significant factor in determining the health of your microbiome is your diet. When we think about foods that are "good for your heart" or "good for your brain" or even "good for your skin," what we might as well be talking about is how good they are for your microbiome. Indeed, your next meal will immediately impact your microbiome and help determine if the good guys are winning or if the bad guys are getting the upper hand.

Fortunately, by choosing to educate yourself about the connection between your gut and your overall health, you've already taken the first step toward changing your life for the better. When you eat well and take care of your body, your microbiome responds quickly; changes in your overall health begin within days.

Yes, it is an exciting time to be a gut doctor. But it's also an exciting time to be a health-conscious person. Because when you understand the work of the microbiome, you understand just how much power you have in your hands to affect the course of your life.

Today is the day to seize that power, to combine ancient wisdom and modern science, and to start taking control over your body, your mind, and your health.

Roshini Raj, MD
Associate professor of medicine, NYU Grossman School of Medicine
Founder of TULA Skincare and cofounder of YayDay
Author, *Gut Renovation: Unlock the Age-Defying Power of the Microbiome to Remodel Your Health from the Inside Out*

Introduction:
You're Not Fat,
You're on Fire!

*A revolutionary way of looking at your body,
and a life-altering plan for feeding it what it
truly needs to stay lean, strong,
and healthy for life.*

YOU ARE NOT "FAT"

No matter what the scale says, no matter what the mirror shows, no matter how you feel when you button your jeans, you are not fat.

In fact, I'm going to go a step further: There is no such thing as a "fat" person.

What we call "fat" is really a symptom of something else. It's your body's response to a chronic underlying health condition that's been linked to everything from cancer to Alzheimer's, from arthritis to diabetes, from heart disease to muscle loss, and, yes, to obesity.

There's a reason why millions of Americans go on diets every year, lose weight, and then see pounds creep back on, often adding even more weight in the process. Because most diets are trying to solve the problem of being "fat." Which is sort of like trying to put out a house fire by turning up the air conditioning. The heat and smoke are just symptoms. What's causing the destruction is the fire underneath.

Most diet programs are trying to cure the symptom. This book will show you how to cure the disease.

And the first step in that process is to stop thinking of yourself as "fat."

When you stop thinking of yourself as fat—and stop buying into the idea that you can change your weight or the shape of your body by going on a diet (read: eating fewer calories), or by exercising more (read: burning off more calories), or by magically changing your metabolism—you can start to address the real issue.

You see, you're not fat.

You're on fire.

A REVOLUTIONARY NEW WAY TO THINK ABOUT OUR BODIES

If this sounds like crazy talk, well, of course it does. You may have been called the F-word in the past, and you've probably used it on yourself as well. But if you were suffering from hay fever, with all its sneezing and sniffling, would you call yourself a "crybaby"? No. It makes no sense to take the symptoms caused by a misfiring of your immune system—symptoms you can't control—and use them to define your body, your lifestyle, or your character.

Yet that's exactly what we're doing when we call ourselves "fat." We're defining ourselves by the symptoms of a chronic autoimmune issue.

That autoimmune issue is inflammation. The remedy for it is in your hands.

And in just the next *seven days*, you're going to take an enormous step toward bringing it under control, with a unique approach that doesn't require calorie restriction, doesn't limit the foods you eat or when you can eat them, and doesn't forbid whole categories of food. Instead, you'll discover how adding more foods into your day—a diverse and delicious array of plants and, yes, even meat and dairy—will help to quell the fire and reset your diet, your health, and your life.

This book will introduce you to a remarkably easy, sustainable, and effective way of eating: *The Full-Body Fat Fix*. This is an anti-inflammation program you can follow for life—one that won't leave you hungry, bored, or feeling like you need to hide under the table when the pizza arrives.

When you control inflammation, you control your destiny. You control your blood pressure, blood sugar, and cholesterol levels; you reduce your risk of Alzheimer's and other brain diseases; you slash your cancer and heart disease risk; and you free yourself from many sources of chronic pain, skin conditions, and autoimmune issues. And, as a side effect, you will see the emergence—the *permanent* emergence—of a leaner, healthier body.

HOW TO SEE YOUR BODY, YOUR DIET, AND YOURSELF DIFFERENTLY

You probably know the allegory of the three blind men trying to describe an elephant. One feels the elephant's side and describes it as "a wall." Another feels its leg and describes it as "a tree." And the third grasps its trunk and exclaims it's like "a snake." They all have pieces of the truth. But none of them has the whole story.

That's how most people, even most experts, approach the issue of weight loss. There are those who see the answer to weight management as resting clearly in low-carb eating, or keto, or calorie restriction, or intermittent fasting, or veganism, or cardio exercise, or some combination of Paleo and CrossFit, or weight-loss surgery, or appetite suppressants, or . . . well, pick your poison. Each of these approaches has its merits, but none illuminates the entire picture, because each is focused on the symptoms. We need to step back and look at the real problem.

And few people have looked at diet, exercise, and weight management from as many different angles as I have. As the author of the *New York Times* bestseller *The Whole Body Reset*, the co-creator of the enormously successful *Eat This, Not That!* franchise, and the editor, writer, and publisher of books and articles on every conceivable diet and fitness program, I've investigated, and, yes, personally tested out, dozens of nutrition and workout plans. I've broken gluten-free bread with tennis star Novak Djokovic and sweated my way through workouts with racecar driver Danica Patrick. In between I've given up sugar, given up meat, given up fat, given up . . . well, just about everything you can give up. And even as I've used my own body as a laboratory, I've stayed on top of the emerging research around fitness and nutrition.

But every piece of information that emerges about health and weight management seems, in the end, to point back to one primary issue—inflammation. And every new approach to eating and exercise nods, to one degree or another, in its general direction. In fact, the primary way any diet or fitness plan works is by reducing inflammation in the body, at least for the short term. And the reason why these plans don't work long-term is that most simply aren't healthy or sustainable, because they don't provide our bodies with enough nutrition to fend off inflammation over the long haul.

The Full-Body Fat Fix presents the first weight-loss program that specifically targets inflammation as the underlying cause of weight dysregulation, and it combines the best aspects of existing weight-management programs with the science and perspective we need to unleash their full potential.

More important, this book is designed to change the way we think about our weight and our health. See, often we make the mistake of thinking that we need to lose weight to be healthier. It's actually just the opposite: We need to be healthier to lose weight. That's why this program is designed to:

- **Stop and Reverse Inflammation** and its many related diseases.
- **Maximize Gut Health** by increasing the biodiversity of your diet.
- **Build and Protect Muscle** through the science of protein timing.
- **Reduce the Risk of Disease** by attacking the primary underlying cause of heart disease, diabetes, Alzheimer's, and other health woes.
- **Lose Weight** without counting calories or cutting out whole food groups.
- **Prevent Frailty** and stay strong, vital, and active.
- **Enjoy Eating** and forget about dieting!

THE REAL GUTS OF THE PROBLEM

When we think about weight issues, we often think about our bellies. But we probably don't think about them in the right way. Because the biggest determinant of whether or not your belly is trying to bust out of your belt buckle is actually hidden deep, deep inside you. It's your microbiome—the approximately 100 *trillion* microbes that call your body home. In fact, only about 10 to 30 percent of the cells in your body are actually human. The other 70 to 90 percent of you is made up of nonhuman microbes. They're on your skin, in your nasal passages, and elsewhere—but the majority of these microbes reside in your large intestine. Do they pay rent? They do not. But they play an enormous role in everything from food digestion to immune system regulation to helping control your mood and energy levels. And current research shows that when it comes to how much you weigh, it's the health of your microbiome—more than how many calories you eat or how often you exercise—that plays the biggest role in determining what numbers show up on the scale.

By the way, about those numbers on the scale: They're not all about you. About five pounds of your overall body weight is actually your microbiome.

And like you, your microbiome gets hungry. But there's a very good chance that you're actually starving your microbiome, by failing to eat enough of the foods those little buggers crave. When we eat processed foods—foods that have been stripped of fiber or otherwise mashed up into an unnatural form—our bodies are able to digest them quickly: think cookies, white rice, white flour, processed meats, fruits that have been ground into "fruit leather," and the vast majority of other foods in the supermarket, most of which come in boxes and bags. That ultra-processed food (or, if you'd like, "predigested" food) is absorbed by our stomachs and small intestines, and never makes its way down into the colon, where the majority of the microbiome lives. In a 2023 study, researchers gave one set of participants a standard Western diet and the other set a diet composed primarily of whole, unprocessed foods—they called that the "Microbiome Enhancer Diet." Both sets of subjects ate the same number of calories per day. The researchers found that when subjects ate whole foods, their microbiomes digested and absorbed an average of 116 additional calories per day. (Some participants lost as much as 400 calories per day to their belly bugs!) But those who ate processed foods wound up absorbing those extra calories themselves.

In other words, your body and your 100 trillion microbial companions are essentially fighting each other for calories. The more whole foods you eat, the more calories your microbiome absorbs and the fewer calories you absorb. This study showed that you could lose weight and body fat simply by switching to a diet that effectively feeds your gut microbes—no calorie-cutting or exercise needed! (And no increase in hunger, either.)

When your microbiome is healthy—when it's in balance, a proper ecosystem with a wide array of different types of bacteria working in concert—then it's more likely that you, too, will be healthy. A healthy microbiome reduces inflammation and our risk of all the diseases, including obesity, that come from it. A 2020 study in the journal *Frontiers in Immunology* pointed to the exact intersection point of gut microbiota, inflammation, and both obesity and type 2 diabetes. The researchers showed how an unhealthy gut triggered inflammation, and how that inflammation led to weight gain and insulin resistance.

Typically, our microbiomes age as we age; researchers have even found that they can tell whether an individual is on the path to frailty by looking at his or her microbiome. But when we keep our gut bugs robust, they keep us robust: A stunning 2023 study of 195 people 100 years old and older living in two "Blue Zones"—Japan and Sardinia— found that the microbiomes of these centenarians were healthier and more diverse than those of younger adults.

What's a "healthy" microbiome? One that includes thriving populations of many different families of microorganisms. The more variety in your microbiome, the less likely you are to be overweight or obese. In one study, researchers compared the microbiomes of seventy-seven sets of twins; they found that the twin with the least variety in his or her microbiome was the one most likely to be overweight or obese.

Remember that word: *variety*. It will be the key factor in how, in just the next seven days, you're going to rebuild your microbiome and start bringing inflammation under control.

VARIETY: THE FOUNDATION OF THE FULL-BODY FAT FIX

In a lot of ways, this program is less like a traditional diet and more like a game—a scavenger hunt or a jigsaw puzzle, perhaps. As you start your journey into the Full-Body Fat Fix—a plant-based, but by no means plant-exclusive, approach to eating—you'll be enjoying plenty of filling and delicious proteins and healthy fats, along with a colorful medley of fruits, vegetables, legumes, nuts, seeds, and grains. You won't be counting calories, restricting whole food groups, or eating in weird time windows or only on certain days. That's not fun.

What is fun is expanding your palate—eating more cool new foods, rather than restricting the ones you love. And expanding our palates—creating more diversity in our daily meals—is crucial. It's the heart of the Full-Body Fat Fix.

Consider this: Only about one in ten of us get enough fruits and vegetables in our diet, according to the Centers for Disease Control and Prevention (CDC). And even if you're in the elite 10 percent who already get at least five servings of fruits and vegetables daily, chances are they're the same fruits and vegetables over and over again: The average American eats about fifty pounds of potatoes a year (think French fries), and about thirty pounds of tomatoes (think pizza and ketchup). After that, onions, carrots, head lettuce (like iceberg), sweet corn, and leaf lettuce (like romaine) are the next five most eaten, but together these five still don't equal our potato total. In fact, by some estimates, 30 percent of the vegetables eaten by Americans are white potatoes.

Our fruit consumption looks pretty much the same: Excluding juices, we eat about fourteen pounds of bananas and ten pounds of apples per year; grapes, watermelon, strawberries, oranges, and pineapple come in at about five pounds or less.

And that's not a natural way to eat. Our bodies are designed to eat a wide variety of plant foods; in fact, scientists discovered in an early

Paleolithic campsite evidence of fifty-five different types of plants—nuts, fruits, seeds, and roots—that our early ancestors had harvested and brought home to eat. That wide variety in the original Paleo diet made for a diverse and healthy microbiome. When another set of researchers compared stool samples from today's humans with remnants of "Paleo feces"—literally, caveman poop—they found that over the past one thousand years the human microbiome has suffered an "extinction level event," losing dozens of species and becoming significantly less diverse. A whopping 39 percent of the microbial species that lived inside us just a few centuries ago are no longer there.

A less diverse diet means a less diverse microbiome, which is one major contributor to many of the diseases of modern humans, including—but hardly limited to—weight gain. Yet most of us—even those of us who try to follow a "healthy diet"— limit ourselves to just a handful of go-tos, especially at breakfast and lunch. In fact, one survey found that one in six people had eaten the same lunch every day for two years. Another found that more than half of Americans eat the same breakfast at least twice a week.

We're all creatures of habit. But *even our healthy habits* can be bad for us if we don't build variety into our routines. It's like if you had the habit of going to the gym every single day, but when you went there you only exercised your forearms. Not only would you *not* look like Popeye, because muscles can only grow in relation to the other muscles that support and surround them, but you'd have strong arms and weak everything else—and be more susceptible to injury, disease, and weight gain. (Not to mention boredom!)

Many of our "healthy" dietary habits have a similar effect. Even if you eat those five servings of fruits and vegetables a day, you're not helping your health to the max unless you're focused on variety: A study at the UC San Diego Center for Microbiome Innovation found that the greater variety of plants your diet holds, the healthier your microbiome. And those with the healthiest microbiomes were people who ate at least thirty different plants a week.

Why is a diverse diet so important? It's hard to know exactly, Daniel McDonald, PhD, a UC researcher on the project, told me recently. One possibility is that, because microbes like to feast on plant fiber, the greater variety is simply healthier for them. Or it could be that certain microbes subsist primarily on certain types of plant fibers, so when we limit the categories of plants we eat, we hinder some aspects of our microbiome and wind up throwing the whole party into chaos.

And it doesn't take long at all for a low-diversity diet to make an impact on our microbiome. Tim Spector, MD, an epidemiology professor at King's College in London, demonstrated this a few years back, when he allowed his son, Tom, to spend ten days eating nothing but McDonald's: chicken nuggets, fries, burgers, and Coke. Before the fast-food fest, Spector took a sampling of Tom's belly biome. Ten days later, he took a second. The result: More than 1,300 specific species of healthy bacteria had been wiped out entirely. Eliminate the variety in your diet, and you eliminate the variety in your microbiome.

There's a second reason why a diverse diet is so much healthier, which has to do with phytochemicals—the unique nutrients found in plants. Each plant has its own set, and there are at least 25,000 different plant-based nutrients that we know of. (That's a lot more than you'll find in even the most comprehensive multivitamin!) Each one of these thousands of nutrients plays a unique role in maintaining overall health: Some have been linked to slowing cognitive decline; others regulate immune system function; still others reduce blood pressure and arterial plaque.

But these diverse nutrients don't work alone. They all work as part of a system, like an orchestra, to create a powerful anti-inflammatory effect. So, if your diet is limited to a routine of potatoes, apples, and broccoli, you're not really feeding your body, or your microbiome, all of the nutrients it needs.

BUT I DON'T WANT TO CHANGE WHAT I EAT!

Yep, roger that. No eating plan is going to work if it doesn't include your favorite foods, or if it involves driving to half a dozen stores trying to find dragon fruit, or kohlrabi, or casaba melon. And not every fruit or vegetable is as universally appealing as watermelon or home fries. That's why making this plan as easy and accessible (and fun!) as possible is so important.

But you also want to see fast results. And that's where the 7-Day Challenge comes in.

What is the 7-Day Challenge? Does it involve eating only avocado for a week? Doing 100 pushups every day? Again, not fun. Instead, the very simple goal of this program is to try to eat thirty different plants in the next seven days. In addition, you'll eat a high-protein breakfast (ideally using whey protein); cut out refined carbs and sweets for just seven days (to jump-start rapid weight loss); and limit your intake of whole grains to one serving per day.

Five Simple Ways to "Cheat" on This Program

Think it's hard to eat thirty plants in one week? Just do this:

- **Turn breakfast into a party.** You don't have to live in Margaritaville to start your day with a frozen concoction. A simple smoothie made with frozen chunks of banana, strawberries, coconut, and mango, plus hemp seeds, ½ a lime, plain yogurt, and vanilla protein powder tastes suspiciously like a daiquiri—and provides you with six Power Plants to start your day.
- **Power up your favorites.** Pasta with marinara sauce has just one whole plant—tomatoes. But use a whole-grain pasta and add some roasted broccoli and fresh garlic, and you just quadrupled the number of plants—while still eating your favorite food.
- **Mix up your greens.** Instead of Bibb, romaine, or iceberg lettuce—or even "superfoods" like kale or spinach—opt instead for the spring mix; you could quadruple the number of plants with this one simple swap!
- **Turn that black bean soup into a twelve-bean soup.**
- **Mix up your nuts.** Instead of a can of peanuts or a bag of pistachios, buy a nut mix that includes almonds, pecans, pistachios, and more. Costco's unsalted nut mix, for example, contains four different plants.

Wait—we got you to thirty different plants just with these cheats alone! And there are plenty of other ways to hit that goal. How about a mixed berry salad instead of just those strawberries? Or a tray of roasted cauliflower, sweet potatoes, and brussels sprouts instead of just one or the other (or the other)? Or sprinkling chia, pumpkin, and sunflower seeds onto your favorite cereal? Or making sure to eat the carrots and celery that come with your chicken wings?

There are a billion different combinations, and this book will show you dozens of paths to hitting your mark. (You'll find fifty more clever ideas on page 17.) But the real cheat is this: Once you spend seven days playing around with this program and challenging yourself to hit your thirty-plant number, you'll have taught yourself how to incorporate plant diversity into your diet. You can start making these choices regularly, expanding your palate, and reaping the benefits for decades to come.

WAIT—IS IT REALLY THAT EASY?

Well, kinda, yeah.

Honestly, if you're already trying to follow a healthy pattern of eating—and not doing something dumb like extreme keto, living entirely on juice, or some other bad-for-you calorie-restriction diet—then you're probably hewing closer to these guidelines than you think. They're based on what we know about the importance of protein, healthy fats, and fiber as the three basic building blocks of human nutrition.

On this plan, you'll eat three meals per day. Your morning meal will be high in protein—aim for 25 to 30 grams—preferably including whey protein or another source of dairy. (I'll explain more in the coming chapters, but protein intake—and especially whey protein—is linked to a healthier microbiome, as well as to muscle maintenance, hunger control, fat loss, higher energy levels, and more.) Most of us already eat plenty of protein at lunch and dinner but fail to start the day properly. That's going to change.

Snacks are optional—the meals in this program are pretty substantial, so you may not find yourself getting hungry at all in between. But when you do nosh, you'll want to put an emphasis on adding more unique plants into your snacking, to ensure that you're reaping the anti-inflammatory, gut-boosting benefits. And, after the initial 7-Day Challenge, you're even going to get a nightly dessert—one that studies show may ward off weight gain and health worries! (I'm not going to keep you in suspense—the dessert-that-makes-you-healthier is on page 48.)

What's great is that you'll be eating plenty of delicious food, with nothing off the table (literally and figuratively) except during your first seven days. And you'll be able to follow this program at many of your favorite restaurants, from Chili's and Applebee's to Subway and Starbucks. Plus, I'll show you dozens of delicious, easy-to-whip-up recipes that will fill your day with Power Plants without making you feel like you're eating like a house finch.

Every meal, and every snack, needs to have all three of the following:

- **Power Plants:** With each plate, you should be building toward your goal of thirty different plants. (Do this and the fiber will take care of itself.) A Power Plant is any whole plant-based food—including grains, nuts, seeds, vegetables, and fruit—that still has its fiber and nutrients intact. A raw apple? Yes. A baked apple? Yes. Applesauce, apple juice, apple fruit leather? No.
- **Power Proteins** (such as plant proteins, lean meats, fish, whole grains, and dairy)
- **Power Fats** (including monounsaturated fats like olives, avocados, and nuts; dairy fats; and fish)

In fact, you can eyeball any meal or snack and ask three questions: Where are my Power Plants? Where are my Power Proteins? Where are my Power Fats? If you know the answer to each of these questions, you know you're on track for a healthy meal, one that will start the process of rebuilding your microbiome, turning down inflammation, and leading you down the path to a leaner, healthier, happier life.

Are you ready to get started?

WAIT, HOLD ON

We need a consensus here. See, you're not embarking on this journey alone. This is a mission for you and the other 100 trillion organisms that make up your body. The whole team needs to work together to quell inflammation, trim fat, and live a longer, healthier, happier life.

So. . . . Is everybody ready? All 100,000,000,000,001 of you?

Then let's go!

The Full-Body Fat Fix at a Glance

Daily Meals: three, including breakfast. Each meal will include 25 to 30 grams of protein, two or more Power Plants, and some form of healthy fat.

Daily Snacks: one or two if you'd like, with at least one Power Plant in each snack.

Key Foods:

Power Plants: as wide an array of whole plants as possible, including nuts, seeds, grains, fruits, vegetables, and legumes. (Every whole, unique plant-based food is a Power Plant!)

Power Proteins: whey protein, lean meats, fish, dairy, poultry, eggs.

Power Fats: olives, avocados, and their oils; nuts, seeds, and their butters; whole-fat dairy; fish.

Foods to Avoid:

- Drinks containing sugar or artificial sweeteners. Studies show that liquid sugar causes profoundly more damage to your body than sugars found in solid food. But weirdly, artificial sweeteners have an almost identical effect. (Read more on page 52.)
- Processed snacks and meals. The more additives, preservatives, and nonfood ingredients we eat, the more we compromise our microbiome. It's impossible to avoid processed foods entirely, but once you make friends with your microbiome, and

understand all that those little buggers are doing for you on a
daily basis, you'll be more thoughtful about protecting them.
• Processed meats. Research shows that many of your favorite
meats—even burgers and steak!—can actually have a protective effect on the microbiome. But processed meats like sausage, bacon, and hot dogs damage the microbiome, increase
inflammation, and increase the risk of obesity, diabetes, and
Alzheimer's disease.

The 7-Day Challenge: For the first seven days, avoid all processed carbohydrates, including white rice, white bread, muffins, cakes, chips,
candy, and so on. Consume thirty different whole plants. Limit whole
grains (such as brown rice and whole wheat bread) to one serving per
day. Give yourself a high five.

50 Ways to Add 100+ Plants

This book is packed with recipes, shopping tips, and even a restaurant guide to help you fill your day—and your digestive system—with an array of inflammation-fighting plants. But there's an unlimited array of ideas for maxing out your plant intake—without having to heat a skillet or pick up a menu. Here are fifty favorites.

1. Amp up your loaf. Try a super-packed multigrain bread like Dave's Killer Bread, which comes loaded with twenty-one different whole grains and seeds including whole wheat, flax, sunflower seeds, sesame seeds, pumpkin seeds, oats, barley, and more.

2. Sneak ground flaxseed into pancake or waffle batter. No one will know!

3. Or steam and purée some cauliflower, and sneak it into pancakes, muffins, even mac and cheese. Again, no one will know!

4. Up your pancake game even more by using buckwheat, a high-fiber, high-protein, gluten-free alternative.

5. Give every smoothie a minimum of six unique plants. (You'll find five recipes to get you started on page 55.)

6. If you're a cereal lover, make a game of topping it with a different fruit, nut, and seed each morning of the week. Strawberries, almonds, and pumpkin seeds today; raspberries, walnuts, and sunflower seeds tomorrow.

7. Speaking of nuts, next time you're hosting a cocktail party, get the nut mix with lots of different nuts, instead of those tired old peanuts.

8. Wait . . . did someone say cocktails? Let's take something

sinful and make it soulful: Muddle some mint for a mojito; use fresh ginger in rum drinks; float some juniper berries in gin. (Just make sure you eat the herbs—no second drink until all the plants are gone.)

9. And if celery garnishes your Bloody Mary, make sure you eat that, too.

10. Wrap your sandwich in cauliflower wraps instead of those sad flour tortillas.

11. Speaking of which, when at a Mexican restaurant, always ask for corn tortillas, which are made from whole grain, instead of flour tortillas, which are just white flour and lard.

12. Never eat ice cream naked. Always top it with nuts and berries (most Froyo joints have plenty of options).

13. And never order a pizza without at least one vegetable topping. Try something new: artichokes, fresh garlic, spinach, broccoli.

14. Check out the new "rice" options, including broccoli, cauliflower, and hearts of palm.

15. Or, instead of plain old white or brown rice, cook up a wild rice blend, which can contain four or five different plants.

16. Play around with new pasta options, including dried pastas made from lentil, chickpea, or brown rice.

17. Or forget about dried pastas altogether and check out alternatives like spaghetti squash or zucchini spirals.

18. Speaking of pastas, you can find frozen raviolis stuffed with spinach, mushroom, eggplant, and squash. Why limit your meal to just one?

19. Check the freezer section for unusual smoothie ingredients—jackfruit, acai, coconut, aloe vera, dragon fruit.

20. Swap that milk chocolate out for a dark chocolate bar that's 72 percent cacao or better.

21. Speaking of chocolate, cacao nibs are broken pieces of cocoa bean that make for fun dessert toppings or even additions to your morning cereal, along with berries and nuts.

22. Find new flours for baking, such as almond, cassava, coconut, chickpea, oat, teff, sorghum, millet, hazelnut, and cauliflower.

23. Up your dipping game with sweet potato chips, plantain chips, or taro chips.

24. And if you're dipping chips, make your own salsa fresca with chopped tomatoes, parsley, onion, seeded jalapeño, and lime juice. Or swap in guacamole or hummus for boring onion dip.

25. Snack on dried seaweed (yes, kids love it, too).

26. Look for alternative crackers like Mary's Gone Crackers, which are made of brown rice, quinoa, pumpkin seeds, sunflower seeds, poppy seeds, and flaxseed.

27. Or forget the crackers altogether and try munching on mushroom crisps or cauliflower crisps.

28. Try Banza mac and cheese—it's mac and cheese made with chickpeas.

29. Look for soup mixes with a wide array of beans and lentils instead of just the same old black bean soup.

30. Pile fresh herbs on top of any fish or chicken you roast in the oven. A little olive oil and salt is all you need to turn it into a flavor explosion.

31. Pour hemp seeds into any smoothie or breakfast cereal. They're loaded with protein, fiber, and healthy fats.

32. Include one piece of fruit every time you have a snack. Craving some cheese? Pair it with an apple. Want chocolate? Cherries or strawberries will go well with that.

33. Give Granny a break. Sure, everyone loves the firm texture and crisp flavor of Granny Smith apples, but there are dozens of varieties to experiment with, and each one is its own plant. Play around with Gala, McIntosh, Fuji, Cortland, Golden Delicious, Pink Lady, and all the other varieties on offer.

34. Same goes for tomatoes—try cherry, beefsteak, plum.

35. Or pears (Bartlett, Bosc, D'Anjou).

36. Look for spring or mesclun mixes in the supermarket, and consider picking up some unexpected salad greens like watercress, sprouts, frisée, and chicory.

37. Move beyond peanut butter and keep almond butter, sunflower butter, and cashew butter on hand as well.

38. Skip the jellies and pick up some of those fancy jams at the farmers market. They're made with whole fruit—you can see the seeds inside—and that counts as a Power Plant.

39. Or go one better and use whole berries with your peanut butter and whole-grain bread. Raspberries and blackberries are especially delicious.

40. When it comes to berries, go wild. Wild blueberries are a dramatically different plant from those raised on farms, and you can find them in the freezer section. Or check out the briar patches in your neighborhood and see if you can track down some wild raspberries or blackberries in summertime.

41. Try unusual nuts like macadamia or Brazil nuts.

42. Use dates to add sweetness. Blended into smoothies or chopped into brownies or muffins, they're a whole-plant alternative to honey or sugar.

43. Skewer your expectations. Instead of plain old steak or chicken, use cubes of meat on skewers with mushrooms, zucchini, tomatoes, even pineapple. (Tip: Soak wooden skewers in water before putting them on the grill to keep them from burning up prematurely.)

44. Make the salad bar your friend. See how many different colors you can fit on one plate. Don't sleep on the beets, radishes, and green beans.

45. Play around with different types of citrus. Instead of just navel oranges, try mandarins, blood oranges, kumquat, tangelo, pomelo—there's a whole world of flavors out there.

46. Pie before cake. Pumpkin, blueberry, apple, peach, cherry . . . anything with a whole fruit in it is a better choice than plain old white flour.

47. Stock your fridge with chia seed pudding. Add chia seeds, a nondairy milk like oat or soy, and a touch of honey. Stir, let sit for ten minutes, then stir again and refrigerate. Serve with chopped fruits on top. It's a breakfast; it's a snack; it's a dessert!

48. When in doubt, get the chili. From Waffle House to Wendy's, plenty of restaurants that seem far from healthy offer plant-rich chilies.

49. Spice up your salad with flowers. Violets and nasturtium are two common edible flowers that seem to grow anywhere. Pick them, let them sit for a few hours on the counter to release any bugs hidden within, and add to your salad or decorate your plate as a garnish. And then . . .

50. Eat the garnish. Whether it's a sprig of mint on a scoop of ice cream, an orange slice on a tequila sunrise, or a frond of parsley on a plate of pork chops, most of us ignore these modest plant offerings—and pass up an opportunity to feed our microbiome what it craves.

1

How Inflammation Makes Us Sick, Bloated, and Unhappy

The Big Bang theory of your belly fat, and why this turning point marks a major change in your life, your health, and your future.

Imagine you've just eaten a filling and delicious meal. You compliment the chef, push back a bit from the table, and place your hand on your belly.

You'll notice that your hand rests comfortably atop your abdomen, right below your chest, a few inches north of your belly button. That resting place is hard, almost ledge-like, with plenty of softer tissue surrounding it.

It may be difficult to remember a time when that swollen lumpiness wasn't there, but your belly is a relatively recent development; you weren't born with it. Your body formed it over time, in response to a slowly smoldering, ongoing health issue you probably have heard about but don't fully understand. That issue is called chronic inflammation. And the center of its universe is your belly. A round gut is the equivalent of a check engine light on your dashboard.

Let's take a look under the hood, and discover exactly what the issue is.

WHAT IS A "LEAKY GUT," EXACTLY?

It seems weird that we can gain weight just because a few trillion microscopic organisms move in one direction or the other. But the balance within your gut can be so delicate that, once it's out of whack (the technical term is "gut dysbiosis"), an extraordinary amount of trouble can occur. Obesity, diabetes, and other disorders are often the result of an inflammation-based issue that doctors call "leaky gut syndrome."

What's that?

Have you ever brushed your teeth and noticed some blood leaking from your gums? That's inflammation—it's caused by a buildup of unhealthy bacteria in and around the space where your teeth meet your gums. As the gums become inflamed, they pull away from the teeth—a condition known as "receding gums"—and more and more of the tooth becomes visible. As the problem gets worse, bacteria and other compounds can enter your bloodstream through these little

What Americans' Finances Tell Us About Fat, Inflammation, and the Calorie Myth

Pop quiz: Which of the following is the best indicator of how much you weigh?

A. Your education level
B. The town you live in
C. The number of cheeseburgers you eat per annum
D. Your hourly pay rate

According to reams of recent research, the answer is All of the Above—except C.

In America, one of the most significant predictors of your weight is your income. In states where median household inleaks in your gums, ratcheting up your inflammation levels. People with gum disease have two to three times the risk of heart attack and stroke as those with healthy gums, and the same bacteria that's found in oral plaque has been found in arterial plaque as well.

Well, what you're seeing in the bathroom mirror when your gums bleed is not unlike what's happening in your gut when your microbiome becomes unbalanced. The lining of your gut becomes inflamed, much like the tissues of your gums. Imagine your gut lining as like a fine mesh, one that allows water and nutrients to flow through, but keeps everything else in its place. As it becomes irritated, the lining swells, and those fine flow points get stretched, creating gaps. At that point, bacteria and their various compounds begin to enter the bloodstream.

One of these compounds, called lipopolysaccharides (LPS), is found in the cell walls of certain bacteria. A healthy gut prevents the flow of LPS into the bloodstream, but a leaky gut lets this compound through. Higher levels of LPS in the bloodstream have been linked to obesity, metabolic syndrome, and inflammation in fatty tissue. In one study, people who were injected with LPS showed an increase in insulin resistance.

comes are below $45,000 a year, more than 35 percent of the population is obese; in states where incomes average more than $65,000 annually, the obesity rate is less than 25 percent. (The same phenomenon is found in Europe, where individuals with lower incomes are up to 20 percent more likely to be obese.)

And this disparity is a pretty recent phenomenon: Researchers at the University of Tennessee, looking at data compiled by the Centers for Disease Control and Food Access Research Atlas project, found that as recently as 1990 there was no discernable connection between income status and obesity. But by 2015, that correlation was undeniable.

I have seen this phenomenon with my own eyes, whenever I drive from New York City to my hometown of Rensselaer, New York, just outside of Albany. It is not what one would call a wildly prosperous community:

This leakage alerts the immune system, which goes into overdrive trying to respond to these unwanted invaders. Meanwhile, the various microorganisms and metabolites begin to collect in the liver, creating damage there, while inflammation grows throughout the body, turning the powerful artillery of the immune system against our own healthy cells, increasing the risk of everything from obesity to diabetes, from heart disease to arthritis.

The good news is that the gut lining is, like most of the rest of our bodies, constantly being regenerated. With a thoughtful, anti-inflammatory, nutrient-packed diet and other lifestyle changes, the gut lining can quickly heal itself—and set you on the path to rapid weight loss.

Median 2020 Property Value, Rensselaer County: $197,100
Median 2020 Property Value, New York County: $1,020,000
Source: Data USA

Motoring up the Thruway with young daughters in tow, I'd have to stop frequently for bathroom breaks, snack breaks, and (for me) coffee breaks. The farther north I got, the heavier the people at the rest stops would be. And when I drove back to the Big Apple, I'd see the phenomenon reverse itself.

Let's stop a minute and think about this. Food costs money. So why does having less money make you gain weight?

One very popular viewpoint is that people with less money are destined to eat the dollar menus at fast-food restaurants, and hence load up on calories. It's a perspective that reached its apogee in the early 2000s, when two teenagers attempted to sue McDonald's for making them obese—just a few short years before the hit film *Super Size Me* landed in theaters. So many, many fast-food calories!

Except when you actually look at the calories fast-food patrons consume, that theory just doesn't hold water:

McDonald's Big Mac, medium fries, and a Coke: 1,040 calories

ANATOMY OF A POTBELLY

Fat is supposed to be our friend.

We may think of the mass in and around our belly as just a collection of unsightly fat cells—also known as adipose cells—but fat is a far more complicated structure. Among those adipose cells are immune cells, which help to clear away pathogens; endothelial cells, which line the blood vessels and help to ensure the flow of nutrients; and nerve cells, which help you feel all the feels. Working together, this collection of cells that form our fatty tissue is the single largest endocrine organ in the body. Every year, about 8 percent of this tissue dies off and is replaced, which means that you get an entirely new set of fat every thirteen years.

Outback Steakhouse cheeseburger, one-half order Aussie fries, and a Coke: 2,290 calories

In fact, while a study of 123 restaurants of every type found that the average meal contained 1,205 calories, Tufts researchers found that the average fast-food meal weighed in at just 809 calories, a remarkable *33 percent less* than full-service restaurants.

The anomaly reaches beyond restaurant culture. Researchers at the University of Minnesota surveyed ninety households within their local community and found that households with higher incomes spent significantly more money both on food served at home and food from restaurants. And they spent more than twice as much money on sweets and snacks than people from lower-income families!

If calories are indeed the driving force in weight gain, then from a purely statistical standpoint, the financially challenged person eating cheap, lower-calorie fast food and saving money on sweets and snacks ought to weigh less than the average well-off American who dines at a wide array of fine eating establishments and doubles down on the Ding Dongs.

Perhaps, then, there's something else at work here.

And when our fat is healthy, these cells all work together to keep us in top shape. The fat cells themselves, teeny-tiny things, secrete a hormone called adiponectin, which does a lot of good stuff: It reduces inflammation, discourages the formation of fatty deposits in the arteries, and enhances the response of cells to insulin, helping to keep blood sugar under control. The immune cells embedded in the fatty tissue contribute to this effort by issuing forth anti-inflammatory compounds of their own. And fatty tissue plays a role in hormonal regulation as well, including estrogen and leptin, the "satiety" hormone that helps to keep hunger at bay.

But when the microbiome becomes disrupted, or when too much fat begins to accumulate, inflammation sets in, and this entire system starts to fall apart. Friend becomes foe. Neighbor turns on neighbor. Fat begets fat.

And the fire begins.

One clue: According to the Minnesota study, while high-income families spent more on junk food, they also spent more than twice as much as poorer families on fresh fruits and vegetables.

That's the disparity. The challenges of fast-food and convenience-food culture don't come from calories; they come from a lack of nutrients, a resulting lack of diversity in the microbiome, and the obesity-promoting inflammation that results. One 2020 study analyzed blood samples from more than 17,000 people and found that, even when accounting for lifestyle factors such as smoking, alcohol use, and BMI, those with lower education levels tended to have higher levels of three markers of inflammation. And in a 2022 study, Harvard researchers found that living in a high-status, high-income neighborhood is associated with lower inflammation.

How strong is the link between financial health, inflammation, and fat? Consider this: Also in 2022, a separate report tracked the increases in visceral fat percentage in the American public between the years 2011 and 2018. Unlike other studies, the researchers in this project sought to look not just at the ongoing increase in people

HOW INFLAMMATION CREATES FAT

You may assume that weight gain means more fat cells, but that's not exactly how it works. Instead, when we take in more calories than we burn, the cells we already have start to swell with stored energy, in the form of triglycerides. This is the kind of weight gain that we might see in early adulthood—a few extra pounds that start to form around our midsection. And it's pretty easy to reverse: If we just eat a little less and exercise a little more, those triglycerides can be burned off, and our fat cells—and our pants—can return to their original size.

A little extra fat is no big deal; indeed, it's natural and maybe even healthy. Studies show that those who gain weight in midlife, but never become obese, live just as long or longer than those who stay lean their whole lives. Remember, fat's job is to protect us.

But there is a tipping point. Researchers writing in the *European*

who were overweight or obese, but at the amount of visceral fat that people were carrying around. They found that, as expected, visceral fat as a percent of body weight continually increased—until 2016. At that moment, the tide seems to have turned, and visceral fat percentage—which is tied directly to inflammation—began to inch downward.

Why? How?

"We had a lot of discussion over why there would be such an inflection point," Jacob E. Earp, PhD, told me. As an assistant professor in the Department of Kinesiology at the University of Connecticut and research associate at UConn's Human Performance Laboratory, Earp was part of the team that conducted the visceral fat study. While they arrived at no definitive explanations, researchers note that this development happens to coincide with two significant changes in American society: a marked downturn in the national poverty rate and widespread enrollment in the Affordable Care Act, leading to a significant reduction in the number of people who were uninsured.

Journal of Immunology called it "the Big Bang": the point at which our fat flips from being a healthy, immune-regulating organ to becoming dysfunctional and dangerous. Whether or not you hit that tipping point depends on the amount of weight you gain, as well as your age, your physique, your level of inflammation, the health of your microbiome, and other aspects of your overall health. But once you do hit it, this additional weight begins to take on a life of its own.

As the adipose cells grow larger—reaching as much as ten times their original volume—they become stressed and produce less of the healthy adiponectin that protects us. Instead, they begin to secrete more pro-inflammatory factors, compounds with ominous, Bond villain–style names like *resistin* and *tumor necrosis factor-a*. The endothelial cells become stressed as well, impairing the flow of oxygen and becoming gummed up with cholesterol. This is a red alert for the

In other words, less poverty + more available health care = less inflammation + less obesity.

But why is a lower income associated with greater fat and higher inflammation? "There's a lot of speculation," Earp told me. "There's discussion about inability to access fruits and vegetables, more reliance on cheaper sources of food—processed food. There's less financial freedom to use recreational facilities. There could be cultural issues as well.

"A lot of it could be the freedom that you have when you don't have as many financial constraints. How much you can spend on produce, how much time you have to go grocery shopping, to cook your own food? If you're working overtime, well, that's time you might have invested into healthy activities." And financial stress, like any other type of stress, is closely linked to rising inflammation. (See Chapter 5: Listening in on the Conversation Between Your Belly and Your Brain.)

But what the evidence tells us is that stress and a lack of dietary variety are significant drivers of obesity. That's why this program isn't about cutting calories and fretting about your weight; it's about kicking back and eating your way lean.

body, which senses real danger as the cells in the fatty tissue struggle for oxygen and nutrients.

As a response, more immune cells—white blood cells called macrophages—begin to form in the fatty tissue. (The heavier you are, the greater percentage of your fat is made up of immune cells. In healthy fat tissue, macrophages make up about 10 percent of the total cells, but as the tissue becomes inflamed, that number can grow to as much as 40 percent. That's right—nearly half of your fat isn't even fat anymore.)

At first, these additional immune cells remain benign. But as the fat mass grows, the immune system panics. The anti-inflammatory cells become outnumbered as more and more inflammatory cells gain purchase, releasing their own Bond-villain compounds. Other cells switch allegiance, like double agents: Invariant-chain natural killer T cells, which work on your behalf to control inflammation when you're lean, suddenly turn on you, flipping into inflammation-promoting mode. The bastards!

These inflammatory compounds spill out into the bloodstream, where they spread throughout the body, inhibiting insulin receptors, further increasing blood sugar levels, and leading to the onset of diabetes. They also affect our leptin receptors; our brains no longer get the signal that we've eaten enough and it's time to stop. Hunger grows. We eat even more.

More food means more blood sugar to deal with. The excess energy is directed right to our bellies.

Fat cells can't duplicate themselves, so, as they fill to the point of overflow, they become even more inflamed, and begin to produce a new hormone, neuropeptide Y (NPY). This hormone signals to stem cells that they need to abandon whatever other plans they had and instead turn into fat cells, increasing the potential storage volume in your belly.

But NPY does something even worse: It is also the most potent appetite-stimulating hormone ever found, acting directly on the brain to make us even hungrier.

Fat begets fat.

This is the inflammation–obesity–hunger cycle that's so difficult to reverse, the one that leads to further weight gain and dramatically increases the prospect of what we call the diseases of aging—heart disease, cancer, Alzheimer's, diabetes, arthritis. A paper published in the journal *Medicine* in 2019 said it plainly: "Obesity is now considered a state of chronic low-grade inflammation."

But all is not lost.

YOUR BODY'S NATURAL FIREFIGHTERS

Our bodies come with a natural defense against chronic inflammation: Among the 100 trillion microorganisms living in your gut are numerous species that work hard to stabilize the immune system, reduce hunger, regulate our hormones, and control inflammation.

They do this in part by breaking down certain types of dietary fiber that our bodies, on their own, simply can't handle. Some species of microbes emit enzymes that help to ferment these otherwise indigestible plant fibers, using them to produce short-chain fatty acids (SCFAs). These SCFAs, as well as other compounds produced by the microbiome, help to reduce inflammation by repairing the gut wall; fighting off invasive, inflammatory bacteria and viruses; producing vitamins; and interacting with a variety of immune-signaling cells. One particular SCFA, called butyrate, has been shown to lower inflammation, improve insulin signaling, promote the breakdown of fat cells—essentially, helping us turn our body fat into energy—and reduce the risk of obesity.

So, in many ways, your gut is populated by trillions of little firefighters, all working to keep inflammation in check—and your belly at bay.

But hidden among the brave heroes in your belly are some arsonists. And when we don't treat our microbiomes right, we feed right into their hands. When our healthy belly bugs don't have enough fiber to chew on, they can't create as many anti-inflammatory SCFAs. That allows more room for unhealthy microbes to grow.

Some of these unhealthy microorganisms create inflammatory compounds, undermining the good works of our benign belly bugs. When these agents of chaos start to take control, they signal our immune systems to rev up unnecessarily. The wall of the gut begins to become irritated, and, as it does so, compounds created by the microbes begin to leak out of the large intestine and enter the bloodstream. Sensing this invasion, the body generates new cytokines to attack these compounds, launching an inflammatory cycle. Meanwhile, immune cells in the lining of the gut come in contact with the bacterial invaders, opening up another front in the war and ratcheting inflammation even higher. Unhealthy gut bacteria can even alter how we extract energy from food—literally making the food you eat more caloric!

As the fire grows, it can start to endanger the very firefighters we're relying on. Inflammation impacts the pH, nutrient availability, and oxygen levels in the gut, effectively snuffing out the helpful microorganisms that want to help you squash the fire while giving more air to the arsonists that are doing the damage.

And this is where our brave belly bugs need our help. The more diverse our microbiome, the more effective it is in helping us fight inflammation. And the number one contributor to gut diversity is our diet; about 57 percent of the variations in our microbiota are determined by what we eat. If we feed them and nurture them, our microbial minions can overcome these challenges and help us overcome our own. In the next chapter, I'll show you how to get started.

An Open Letter from Your Microbiome

Take a peek in any supermarket, drugstore, or vitamin vendor, and you'll see there's no shortage of savvy supplement salesmen ready to sell you something that's healthy for your microbiome. But do any of the many, many products marketed as "probiotic" actually make a difference? We decided to go right to the source. We asked your belly bugs what really makes them happy, and they answered with one voice. (Okay, with 100 trillion teeny-tiny voices.) Here's their advice to you.

Dear Host Human,

Greetings from the depths of your cecum!

Did you not know you had a cecum? You do: It's the little pocket at the entryway to your large intestine, where the vast majority of us reside. Sure, there are a handful of yeasts, lactobacilli, and streptococci that flourish in your stomach, and some additional bacteria strains in the small intestine as well. But the real party is here, in the cecum. It's like the Ibiza of your intestines.

Anyway, we're reaching out to thank you for taking such an interest in us, but also to share some advice on those "good for your gut" products—the ones that make us happy, the ones that make us mad, and the ones that just make us go, Hmmmm. Here's a look at which products are worth purchasing—and which you should take a pass on.

BELLY GOOD: Plain yogurt and kefir. Yogurt and kefir are fermented, which means they're dense in probiotics like S. thermophilus and B. lactis. And we like those guys. In fact, a 2022 study in BMC Microbiology found that yogurt consumption "is associated with reduced visceral fat mass and changes in gut microbiome." Greek yogurt is higher in protein than regular yogurt, by the way, and hence better at helping you burn fat and hold on to muscle.

BELLY BAD: *Flavored yogurts, "fruit on the bottom" yogurts, and yogurt drinkables.* When you add sugar to a yogurt or yogurt drink, all bets are off—the sugars feed your bad bacteria, the bullies who want to colonize your gut and keep it for themselves. For example, Chobani Low-Fat Plain Greek Yogurt has 4 grams of sugar per ¾ cup serving—the natural sugar that's found in dairy. But a container of Chobani Low-Fat Passion Fruit on the Bottom Greek Yogurt has 14 grams of sugar! Check out the ingredients: Cane sugar is number three on the list, along with locust bean gum. I mean, who doesn't love a good locust bean? But, come on—added sugars and preservatives do more harm than the yogurt does good.

BELLY GOOD: *Fresh sauerkraut and kimchi.* Stanford researchers recently put two groups on special diets. One ate a lot of fiber, and one ate primarily fermented foods, such as kimchi. Researchers found that eating fermented foods "enhances the diversity of gut microbes and decreases molecular signs of inflammation" even more so than a high-fiber diet does. Look for little bubbles in the liquid, which is a sign of fermentation, and the words *lacto-fermented* and *unpasteurized*.

BELLY MEH: *Shelf-stable sauerkraut and kimchi.* Here's the thing: The fermented foods we like are the ones that need to be kept cold. So, if you buy it out of the refrigerator case, you're probably in good shape. But shelf-stable foods that you can find on the shelves and store in your pantry before opening? They've been pasteurized, meaning all the bacteria—healthy or not—has been wiped out. A microbial massacre! We still appreciate the fiber and other nutrients in pasteurized foods like these. But you can do better.

BELLY BAD: *Kombucha tea.* It's bubbly; it's trendy; it's got just a tiny bit of alcohol, so it's a little naughty. But for all its probiotics, kombucha has one problem: It's loaded with sugar, often to the tune of 14 grams of added sugar per serving. (That's about one and a half glazed doughnuts' worth, or more than a third of the total added sugar the American Heart Association says a person should consume in a given day.) No amount of probiotics is worth all that sugar cane raising Cain!

BELLY BAD: *Probiotic supplements.* There are three reasons why probiotic pills are potentially problematic—and not particularly potent.

They aren't regulated: Supplements typically list colony-forming units (CFUs) on their labels, a measure of microbial mass. But the CFU might not be accurate (supplements aren't regulated the way drugs are). Or it might be the total mass of both live and dead probiotics—and only the live ones make any difference. After a stay on the drugstore shelf and another tour of duty in your pantry, there's no telling if the CFUs are DOA.

Your stomach is like a lake of fire; almost nothing survives in there. So, left naked and unshielded by food, most of the bacterial species that do make it alive into your belly will be quickly destroyed—and remember, you want those bacteria to get all the way through the stomach, through the small intestine, and down here to the colon—party central.

Probiotic pills don't contribute variety. Even the best supplement, one with really robust CFUs and an enteric pill coating that helps it survive the stomach acid, only comes with a handful of different types of microbes. So even if you deliver the goods, alive and kicking, all the way to the cecum, you're probably not doing a whole lot to increase the variety of microbes in your gut. A recent study looked at people taking antibiotics; those in the control group, who just took the antibiotics, saw their microbiomes rebound back to normal within three weeks. But the microbiomes of those who took probiotics in addition to antibiotics had still not returned to normal after five months, and showed less microbial diversity!

Bottom line: You've got 100 trillion fans rooting for you. But we can't keep you healthy unless you keep us healthy. More fiber, more fermented foods, less sugar, and fewer weird chemical thingies, please. Remember: We're all in this together.

Best,

Your Belly Bugs

Extra-Delicious Special Section

The Fire-Fightin' Five!

Is there such a thing as a "perfect" day of eating? One that feeds your microbiome and lowers your inflammation levels so effectively it couldn't possibly be improved on? Probably not. But this is as close as you can get. These five recipes—a breakfast smoothie, a sandwich for lunch, a pizza appetizer, a pasta dinner, and a dessert—will provide you with somewhere between thirty and forty different plants in a single day, as well as the optimum doses of protein and calcium you'll need throughout to keep your muscles and bones strong.

Should you eat this menu every day? No freakin' way! Because each meal ought to be a fun scavenger hunt for more unique fruits, vegetables, nuts, seeds, and grains to add into your day. But it just goes to show how simple it is to get to thirty plants—and beyond!

Breakfast
Kale to the Chief protein smoothie (recipe, page 58)
A blend-it-in-seconds morning drink packed with protein and fiber.
Power Plants: kale, parsley, oats, flaxseeds, date, chia seeds

Lunch
Steak Sandwich with Aioli (recipe, page 186)
Pile a whole-grain hoagie roll with leftover protein and tons of sautéed veggies. So simple!
Power Plants: Multigrain bread (whole wheat and others), portobello mushroom, red bell pepper, red onion, mesclun greens (may include plants such as spinach, green leaf lettuce, baby romaine, mustard greens, and so on), kalamata olives, dill

Appetizer

Perfect Pizza (recipe, page 189)

A make-it-in-minutes crowd pleaser you can whip up using premade crusts (or follow the recipe if you want to do it from scratch).

Power Plants: San Marzano tomatoes, basil, oregano, figs, arugula

Dinner

Totally Tubular Pasta with Grilled Chicken (recipe, page 188)

A simple pasta piled high with vegetables and lean grilled chicken.

Power Plants: Vidalia onion, garlic, eggplant, zucchini, shiitake mushrooms, Thai bird's eye chili, rosemary, chives

Dessert

Berry Good Ricotta (recipe, page 213)

It tastes like ice cream but has the muscle-building power of a protein drink.

Power Plants: strawberries, blueberries, cherries, peaches, mint

2

The Full-Body Fat Fix in Three Simple Steps

Understanding Power Plants, Power Proteins, and Power Fats, and the role that each plays in our overall health system. Plus: Why "superfoods" are actually kryptonite.

America has a diversity problem.

It's not in our magnificent melting pot, or in the beautiful array of individuals who make up our nation. The diversity problem facing America is one that's found deep inside us as individuals. It's a lack of variety in our diets and a lack of variety in our microbiomes.

And it helps to explain why the United States is, in many ways, unique in its obesity challenge: We get nearly 60 percent of our daily calories from ultra-processed foods, according to a study in *BMJ*. (The only other country in the world that gets more than 50 percent is the United Kingdom, according to a meta-analysis of 100 studies around the globe.) By comparison, people in Italy eat less than 10 percent of their daily calories from these products. And remember, the more ultra-processed foods we eat, the more calories we absorb— and the fewer calories get taken up by our microbiomes.

Now consider that more than 36 percent of the U.S. population is obese—the highest in the world among major countries. In Italy, that number is less than 20 percent. In China, it's 6 percent.

It's the uniqueness of our American diet that's causing so much havoc on our microbiomes, damaging our belly bugs' natural ability to fight inflammation and keep obesity at bay. In this chapter, we'll start the process of coming to their rescue—so they can come to ours.

THE PROBLEM WITH PROCESSING

What are "ultra-processed foods"? Ultra-processed foods contain stuff that we don't think of as food—artificial preservatives and colors, hydrogenated fats, emulsifiers, cellulose—or else things that once were parts of foods but have been extracted and altered, such as added sugars, weird-sounding starches, and fats from places we don't think fat should come from (like corn, palm trees, and whatever a canola is). Essentially, any food that has an ingredient that you can't draw a mental picture of (what does xanthan gum look like?) is an ultra-processed food. And ultra-processed foods are foods that have, in most cases, been stripped of their diverse plant fibers and phytonutrients. They've been made to conform.

Of course, we all know how addictive ultra-processed foods are. "Bet you can't eat just one" is a tagline for a reason: These foods are literally engineered to make it hard for us to eat in moderation. And because things like cookies, crackers, candy, chips, fast food, and sweetened breakfast cereals are dense in calories, we wind up overeating without even realizing it. Ultra-processed foods are generally low in fiber and protein, so we don't get that satisfied feeling we should get after eating, while some contain additives that can interfere with our hormones or trigger our brain's reward center, making it hard to stop eating once we start.

But these sneaky snacks have another serious side effect: They're really, really good at creating inflammation. One 2022 study found that the more ultra-processed foods people ate, the higher their blood levels of inflammatory compounds like C-reactive protein and tumor necrosis factor-a.

How do these foods cause our inflammation levels to spike? One way is by disrupting our microbiomes. Some food additives, such as emulsifiers (lecithin, polysorbates, carrageenan, guar gum, monoglycerides, and diglycerides) have been shown to directly alter the gut microbiome, as have sugar and artificial sweeteners (see Sweet and Lowdown, page 52). Another way is by flooding our bodies with too much sugar and too little fiber, causing a race to store calories in our fatty tissues. The third way is by taking up space in our tummies that should be filled by a wide, diverse array of whole foods, especially plants. And a fourth way is that, because they are absorbed high up in the digestive tract, they wind up starving our microbes of the energy they need—while putting all those empty calories right into our own bodies!

All of this creates a crisis in our bellies. The Full-Body Fat Fix is here to help. To follow the Full-Body Fat Fix, you need only to answer these three questions:

Where are my Power Plants?

Where are my Power Proteins?

Where are my Power Fats?

If you imagine a plate, it should be made up of about three-fourths Power Plants and about one-fourth Power Proteins. Most of those Power Plants should be fruits, vegetables, nuts, and seeds, accompanied by a smaller amount of whole grains and legumes. The Power Fats are the finishing touch, as you'll see below.

Here's how the components work and how to build, buy, or order the perfect meal for you.

POWER PLANTS FOR A FLAT BELLY

The basics: Each meal should have at least two different Power Plants. Aim for thirty different Power Plants every week.

What makes a plant food a Power Plant? It's pretty simple, really.

It's an actual plant—or at least the root, stem, leaf, fruit, or seed of a plant. One that grows. In the ground.

Even as we learn more and more about the value of whole foods, as a society we seem determined to find ways to avoid eating them. Driven by a fascination with technology and a desire for convenience, we've been striving for the past hundred years to turn our world into something that resembles an episode of *The Jetsons*: We all want to come home from a long day's work at Spacely Sprockets, dock the flying car, hand our coat to Rosey the Robot, and tuck into a delicious meal straight from the Food-a-Rac-a-Cycle.

While flying cars and robotic handmaids aren't yet a thing, we're already summoning just about any food we want from push-button devices. And I'm not just talking about the microwave. Dessert toppings like edible wedding cake toppers are often now 3D printed; printed pizza is in development; and there's even a machine called the PancakeBot that automatically creates pancakes in whatever shape you can imagine.

Yet our race to create new stuff we can put into our mouths is moving us further and further from what we know as food—no matter how much manufacturers want us to think otherwise. Case in point: the rise of "whole food supplements." Products like Balance of Nature Fruits & Veggies claim to deliver the nutrition found in dozens of different plants in the convenience of a pill, while powders like AG1 are a mix of "superfoods" condensed down into a powder you can mix with water. "It's all you really need, really," says AG1's marketing materials.

Well, no, not really. While these products may or may not deliver vitamins, minerals, and phytonutrients, what they're not capable of delivering are the unique plant fibers that are so critical to our microbiomes. AG1 claims it gives you twelve servings of fruits and vegetables in one glass. But that glass will provide just 2 grams of fiber, about half of what you'd get if you just ate an apple.

So, eat the apple. Pills and powders don't count. (You'll read more about why in Chapter 7: Put Those Damn Vitamin Pills Down—Now!)

Fruit and vegetable juices, even ones you squeeze at home or pick up at the New Age juice bar, don't count either, for the same reason: Once a plant is pressed into a juice, it's stripped of the fiber your microbiome needs. (And fruit "pulp" can only make up a tiny bit of the difference.) A cup of fresh-squeezed orange juice has less than ½ gram of fiber, while a cup of whole orange segments gives you seven times as much.

Here are the general rules for Power Plants:

- Each plant must be the whole plant, or the edible part of the plant, with its fiber or nutrients still intact. That means that Doritos don't count as corn, sourdough doesn't count as wheat, and Uncle Ben's doesn't count as rice. But popcorn counts, and so does whole wheat bread and brown rice. Fruits, roots, nuts, seeds, flowers, leaves, stems—these are the hallmarks of the Power Plants.
- Fruits and vegetables that are whipped up in a blender or food processor still count, as long as you're still eating the whole plant. But juices don't count, as the fiber has been almost entirely removed.
- Plant "milks" don't count. Almond milk is the nutritional equivalent of water, except in cases where it's been fortified.
- Herbs and spices don't count, unless you're eating enough that it would be equivalent to eating, say, a salad component—at least one-eighth of a cup of fresh sprigs. So a parsley or basil pesto would be a Power Plant, and some of the smoothie and salad recipes you'll see in this book include herbs among the Power Plants because I use at least one-eighth of a cup in each recipe. But sprinkling some dried basil onto your omelet doesn't meet the mark.
- Granny Smith, Fuji, Red Delicious—each variety counts as a Power Plant. Yes, they're all apples, but "while they share a common ancestry, they have different phytochemical makeup," Jim Germida, PhD, emeritus professor in the Department of Soil Science at the University of Saskatchewan, Canada, told me recently. Indeed, all plants have distinct microbiomes of their own, which live both on them and within them, says Germida. The same is true for different varieties of grapes. As for peppers: Red and green bell peppers are the same plant (the red ones are just ripened, and hence more nutritious). But jalapeños, banana wax, shishito, and cherry peppers all count as separate plants. And those of you who are really up on your plant biology know

that broccoli, cauliflower, kohlrabi, cabbage, kale, and brussels sprouts are all descendants of the same plant—the wild mustard. But each counts as its own separate Power Plant.

POWER PROTEINS FOR A LEAN, STRONG BODY

The basics: Every meal should have 25 to 30 grams of protein. Make protein in the morning a priority.

Imagine a plate of spaghetti and meatballs. Hold off on the parmesan, just for a moment.

Let's say, for argument's sake, that on that plate was about 600 calories' worth of protein—primarily from the meatballs, although the pasta has some too—and another 600 calories from the pasta and the sauce. So, 1,200 calories in all. (It's a big plate.)

You'd think that eating those 1,200 calories of spaghetti and meatballs would mean 1,200 calories added to your daily bottom line. But here's where the whole idea of dieting based on cutting calories starts to fall apart.

See, when you eat carbohydrates, somewhere between 5 and 10 percent of your total calorie intake is burned away by what's called the "thermic effect of food" (TEF). TEF measures the increase in calorie burn inside your body caused by the effort it takes to digest that food. So when you eat 600 calories of carbs, you're really only getting between 540 and 570 calories.

But what about that meatball? Incredibly enough, the TEF of protein is somewhere between 20 and 30 percent—or three to four times higher. So your 600 calories of meatball translates to just 400 to 480 calories. The higher the percentage of protein on your plate, the lower your final calorie total might turn out to be.

And the greater your potential for lean muscle mass and less fat. As you'll read further in the coming chapters, we begin to lose the ability to turn protein into muscle as early as age thirty, and the problem only accelerates with age. When we get older, we need to have larger doses of protein; depending on your body size, it takes about 25 to 30 grams of protein at one meal to turn on the processes that help us build and maintain muscle. So it's important that each meal contains adequate protein so that we continue to build and maintain muscle throughout the day.

The critical meal is breakfast; that's when the average American awakens from ten or more hours of not eating and then sits down with, on average, a mere 10 grams of protein—not nearly enough to jump-start the muscle-making process. Protein for breakfast is make-or-break time for your muscles.

If protein is so great, shouldn't we all be on a high-protein diet?

Well, no. While it is crucial to have adequate protein throughout the day, more in this case is not better, because study after study has shown that while high-protein diets do increase the number of microbes in our guts, they have an overall negative effect on microbe diversity. And diversity is what we are after.

The key is moderation. Most of us eat about twice as much protein as we need at dinner—an average of 60 grams every night. Instead, we want to spread our protein throughout the day, a technique known as *protein timing*. And it's here, too, where the notion of diversity continues to matter.

Different types of protein—even when they're from the same animal—affect the microbiome in unique ways. Our guts respond differently to egg protein than to chicken protein; differently to dairy than to beef. And in animal studies, mice fed a mix of protein sources showed more diverse microbiomes than those who consumed only casein-based protein.

Yet while a mix of different proteins—including dairy, red meat, poultry, fish, and plant-based protein—probably makes sense, there is one type of meat that has been shown to be very, very bad for your microbiome: processed meat. Sausage, bacon, hot dogs, cold cuts—for as long as you plan to make your microbiome your friend, these should be off your plate. In fact, a large study of more than 490,000 people published in the *American Journal of Clinical Nutrition* found that for every ounce of processed meat in your daily diet, your risk of Alzheimer's disease increases by 52 percent. The reason: Processed meat damages your microbiome, raising your inflammation levels. (Interestingly, in the same study, while fresh poultry had no effect on a person's risk for dementia, unprocessed red meat—beef, lamb and pork—was shown to actually *lower* dementia risk. So, hamburger—yes; hot dog—no.)

POWER FATS FOR SUPER NUTRITION

The basics: Each meal should have at least one source of healthy, nutritionally dense fat, which could include dairy, omega-3 fatty acids from seafood, or other monounsaturated fats from nuts, seeds, olives, or avocado.

If you pay any attention to diet trends, you know that keto diets have been extremely popular over the past few years. A keto diet is one that is super low in carbohydrates, moderate in protein, and very high in fat; the idea behind the keto diet is to prevent your body from using glucose—which your body makes from carbohydrates—as energy, instead burning fat preferentially, a state known as "ketosis." (Because the body can convert protein into glucose, even muscle-building proteins are limited on a keto program.) Supermarkets and drugstores are filled with "keto-friendly" snacks and "fat bombs" designed to flood your body with fat to suppress your hunger and keep you from eating any carbohydrates.

Are "fat bombs" good for your microbiome? No.

One study followed 217 people for six months and found that those who ate a diet that was 40 percent fat created unhealthy changes in the microbiome, while diets lower than that threshold seemed to create a healthier belly environment. (A strict keto diet, for reference, is usually north of 50 percent of calories from fat, and can be much higher.)

What about low-fat diets—the craze of the 1990s? Again, no. Fat in moderation is good for your microbiome, and for you overall. Fat is crucial for brain function—the brain is nearly 60 percent fat. Fats are crucial for helping our bodies digest and process the nutrients in our food, especially the fat-soluble vitamins A, D, E, and K. Monounsaturated fats like seeds, nuts, olives, and avocado—and their spreads and oils—and omega-3 fatty acids found in seafood as well as chia seeds and flaxseeds specifically help to reduce inflammation. And because inflammation is the chief mischief maker within the body, it makes sense that these fats have also been shown to lower the risk of heart disease, diabetes, dementia, and a wide array of other health issues.

But you don't need to limit yourself just to these plant-based options. A recent review of studies found that, for the most part, changing up the fat in your diet doesn't have a significant impact on the microbiome. While there are some indications that a diet high in saturated fat (typically found in animal products) may have some negative impact on microbiome diversity, the findings have been inconclusive.

In fact, the idea of one or more types of fat being a cure-all (think monounsaturated fats or omega-3s) or a singular evil (think saturated fat) has been pretty well debunked. While it was commonly believed that some fats were bad for your heart and others were good for it, a review of studies in the journal *Nutrients* in 2021 found that "the matrix effect"—essentially the overall content of your diet—seems to be the principal determinant of the connection between dietary fat, inflammation, and cardiovascular disease. In other words, we don't need to worry about fat as much as we've been told, as long as we eat a balanced diet filled with healthy foods that provide a wide array of nutrients.

The ideal fat source, then, is one that delivers the most nutrients. Fats like vegetable oils—canola oil, corn oil, palm oil, or soybean oil—are highly processed, condensed down to a low-nutrient state. That processing results in these fats carrying an unusually high level of linoleic acid, which has been linked to increased inflammation. (Because these oils are cheap, they're what restaurants like to fry stuff in. As a result, the average American eats 3 tablespoons of vegetable oil every day, most of it from fast food or processed foods.)

Fats that are closer to the actual food source they come from—dairy fats, for instance, or the fats that occur naturally in fish and meat, or those that are pressed from nuts, seeds, and fruits like olives and avocados—carry a much higher nutritional payload. Animal fats deliver essential amino acids and, through dairy, bone-strengthening calcium. Nuts and seeds deliver a wide array of vitamins and minerals, especially vitamin E. Olive oil is rich in two unique phytochemicals (hydroxytyrosol and oleocanthal) that have anti-inflammatory properties. (When you taste an extra-virgin olive oil and feel that slight burn at the back of your throat, you're tasting the oleocanthal; the purer the olive oil, the more burn you'll feel—and the more protective phytochemicals you're enjoying.)

Each meal on the Full-Body Fat Fix should include at least one of these healthy fats. And of course, fatty plants like nuts, seeds, and their butters, as well as olives and avocados, count toward your Power Plant total. Oils, on the other hand, don't: While avocado oil and olive oil—especially extra-virgin olive oil—are closely linked to lower inflammation and positive health outcomes, to count as a Power Plant you need to eat the whole plant, fruit, seed, root, or flower, and hence that plant's unique fiber content. So maybe there's some tapenade or guacamole in your future?

Can This Dessert Save Your Life?

Cutting down on sugar—especially during the 7-Day Challenge, which we will discuss in the next chapter—isn't just part of this program. It's part of just about every healthy eating program ever developed.

Still, the tongue craves sweetness. We evolved in a time of limited resources, competing for calories and nutrients with bears, monkeys, raccoons, and other mammals, as well as just about every other creature that walked, crawled, or flew about the earth. So it made sense that we also evolved to crave sweets; naturally occurring sugars in fruits made these items particularly tasty, and fruits are loaded with nutrients our bodies need. A primitive tribe that came across a tree heavy with dates or figs would gather, and eat, everything they could get their hands on, because if they didn't pig out, some other animal (or tribe) would get the goods.

Today, we don't have to hike across the desert looking for dates and figs to satisfy our sweet tooth. We just have to go to the supermarket. Or the gas station. Or the movie theater. Or the hardware store, the office supply outlet, the pharmacy . . . you name it. Pretty much anywhere that money changes hands, a crafty marketer has placed sweets for sale near the checkout counter, luring us in with those intuitive survival instincts we developed millennia ago.

And sweets are bad for us. Except, maybe . . .

Ice cream.

Study after study has shown that people who consume more dairy, particularly yogurt, have a lower risk of developing diabetes. But among that data was another surprising finding: The same studies found that men who had at least two half-cup servings of ice cream per week also had a lower risk of diabetes. And a 2018 Harvard study found that among diabetics a half cup of ice cream per day was associated with a lower risk of cardiovascular disease.

What's going on here?

First of all, there are the benefits of dairy, which you'll read about throughout this book: It's filled with protein, particularly the amino acid leucine, which helps build and maintain muscle. It also delivers calcium, vital to regulating blood pressure and preserving bone health. So a little bit of ice cream does, indeed, pack a bit of a health punch.

Second, there's the fact that if you're eating ice cream, you're probably not eating something else for dessert: cookies, candies, cake, pastries, and other foods that deliver all of that sugar but no protein or other nutrients. In fact, the glycemic index—a measure of how much a food spikes your blood sugar levels—is actually lower for ice cream than it is for many healthy carbs such as brown rice.

So: Dessert isn't a requirement of this program, and sugar is an evil you should avoid as much as you can (and swear off of entirely during the 7-Day Challenge). But if your sweet tooth is acting up at night, I strongly encourage you to satisfy it with a little ice cream. You might actually be doing your health some good!

DEATH OF THE SUPERFOODS

Throughout this book, I'm talking a lot about plant and dietary diversity. What I'm not talking about is what every other nutrition hype machine seems obsessed with: superfoods.

To understand the concept of superfoods, let's take a trip back in time to your childhood home. Think back to the sights and sounds and smells of your parents' house at dinnertime. Maybe Dad is in the backyard, spatula in hand, yellow flames sizzling up off the grill, putting the final touches on a chunk of seitan to serve with his special side salad of kale, quinoa, and goji berries. Mom might be in the kitchen, whipping up one of her delicious chia seed, acai, and spirulina puddings. Can you still remember the smell of coconut oil wafting through your family kitchen?

No? No, no, and no?

Today, no progressive pantry or trendy smoothie and salad bar would be complete without most, if not all, of these "superfoods," along with matcha powder, hemp seeds, kamut, fenugreek, turmeric, stinging nettles, and maybe a sprouted mung bean or two. In fact, by 2030 the "global superfoods market" is forecasted to reach $246.2 billion.

That's a lot of sprouted mung beans.

And yet, few if any of these foods were even on our radar thirty years ago. Where did they all come from? Why are our supermarkets now populated by plants and products that sound more like minor Avengers characters than like something we'd want to put in our mouths?

These exotic foods join a more recognizable collection of things we used to eat once in a while but have since been elevated to superhero status: blueberries, salmon, Greek yogurt, avocados, walnuts, olive oil. In fact, if you read pretty much any diet book or nutrition plan written over the past twenty years, it was likely that you came across a page, early in the program, with a chart of "superfoods" that were selected as the "secret weapons" to "power up" your diet.

What makes a particular food qualify for elevation to Marvel Universe stardom, other than being exotic/expensive/weird tasting? One traditional way for foods to get the superhero status is known as the ORAC score. The National Institutes of Health ranks foods according to this score (ORAC stands for Oxygen Radical Absorbance Capacity, which again sounds like something Iron Man uses to power his suit). The higher a food's ORAC score, the more antioxidants it contains: Prunes, raisins, blueberries, blackberries, kale, spinach, and raspberries top the USDA's list.

Typical "superfoods."

If you've been a health-conscious person over the past forty years, but especially in the 1990s, you probably heard an awful lot about how free radicals—rogue oxygen molecules—caused aging, and how antioxidants—vitamins C, A, and E, in particular—were the key to beating back the tides of time. You might have even taken daily doses of them. This was known as "the free-radical theory of aging," which was first posited back in 1956.

Have you noticed that you haven't heard much about free radicals lately? That's because the reality of free radicals has in many ways proven far more complicated than we've been told. A meta-analysis of more than five hundred studies found that while high levels of these molecules can be damaging, more moderate levels actually retard aging and protect us against disease.

But as the idea of antioxidants and the importance of ORAC scores have faded, plenty of other foods have been held up as "superfoods," even by prestigious organizations. The Cleveland Clinic's *Health Essentials* newsletter lists fourteen superfoods: avocado; berries; beets; chia seeds; cinnamon; dark, leafy greens; garlic; ginger; green tea; lentils; pumpkin; salmon; yogurt; and kefir. The *Harvard Health Blog,* on the other hand, has ten: Like the Cleveland Clinic, they include berries, fish, leafy greens, yogurt, and legumes (which includes lentils), but then they have tomatoes, cruciferous vegetables, whole grains, olive oil, and nuts. The wellness website Everyday Health nominates pomegranate, citrus fruits, kimchi, and "ancient grains."

The problem with the "superfoods" concept is that it leads us to believe that if we just eat plenty of wild blueberries, or organic teff, or spirulina smoothies, we're going to be in great shape. And so we focus in on these specific foods, adding them into our day whenever possible—sometimes to the exclusion of more mundane fare like oranges or whole potatoes or watermelon, which have their own unique set of nutrients. A handful of goji berries can't compare to the nutritional impact of a handful of mixed berries; lentil soup just isn't as powerful as a chili made with many different types of legumes and vegetables.

Here's the truth: There is only one superfood out there. It's whatever plant food you're *not* eating.

Sweet and Lowdown

We all know that there's a link between excessive sugar consumption and weight gain. Must be the calories, right? But there's also a link between artificially sweetened, zero-calories drinks and weight gain, too. How can this be? How can the calories in soda and the complete lack of calories in diet soda have the same effect?

Because it's not the calories.

Do calories matter? Of course. But they're just one contributing factor. As we'll see throughout this book, there are a lot of different factors that go into that number on the scale, and calories is just one of many. And nowhere is that fact made clearer than in the comparison between calorie-loaded sugary drinks and calorie-free, artificially sweetened drinks. Consider:

- **Sugar damages the microbiome**. A diet high in sugar has been shown to decrease gut biodiversity and promote inflammatory gut microbes, essentially helping them to take over and squash their anti-inflammatory belly mates. Specifically, sugar seems to damage a type of bacteria called *Bacteroidetes*, which has been linked to leaner, flatter bellies, and boost the bacterium *Proteobacteria*, which in moderate amounts is part of a healthy microbiome, but when it grows out of control, it has been linked to greater inflammation and weight gain. Sugar also damages the lining of the gut, inflaming it and creating a greater likelihood of leakage.

    ◊ **But so do artificial sweeteners.** A study of aspartame, saccharin, and sucralose found that the sweeteners seemed to enhance the ability of unhealthy gut bacteria, including E. coli, to invade and damage the lining of the intestinal wall, leading to leaky gut, while making it harder for healthier and more diverse microbes to sustain themselves. And saccharin has been shown to alter the gut microbiome in a way that promotes diabetes.

- **Sugar boosts inflammation and increases the risk of disease.** Excessive sugar intake has been linked to heart disease, high blood pressure, high cholesterol, stroke, diabetes, autoimmune disease, and obesity—all diseases that are tied directly to our inflammation levels. One study found that blood levels of the inflammatory marker C-reactive protein spiked after subjects drank a fluid containing 50 grams of sugar. (For reference, a grande Mocha Frappuccino from Starbucks has 51 grams.) Another study found that just one sugary soft drink per day raises your risk of metabolic syndrome (a combination of obesity, high cholesterol, and high blood sugar) by 44 percent.

    ◊ **But so do artificial sweeteners.** In fact, eating or drinking artificial sweeteners has been linked to an increase in inflammatory bowel disease (IBD) and other inflammatory conditions because of the changes that they cause in our gut biology. A study of 3,000 people found those who consumed the highest levels of erythritol, a sugar alcohol that's used as a sweetener in many "keto-friendly" foods, were about twice as likely to have a "cardiovascular event" (read: heart attack or stroke) as those who consumed the least. Another study, from 2023, looked at more than 103,000 people and found that sucralose and acesulfame potassium (Ace K) were both associated with an increased risk of heart disease, while aspartame was linked to a greater risk of stroke. These two sweeteners in particular have also been linked to an increased risk of breast cancer and obesity-related cancers.

- **Sugar forces the growth of new fatty tissue in the gut.** As I explained in Chapter 1, belly fat is made up of fat cells as well as immune cells. When we consume sugar, the inflammation-friendly immune cells in our guts become activated, resulting in an even greater increase in inflammation, hunger, and visceral fat.

    ◊ **But so do artificial sweeteners.** In fact, artificial sweeteners cause weight gain by increasing hunger through a number of different pathways. Researchers in Australia noticed that animals who were exposed to high levels of artificial sweeteners ate more than those who were not. They found that sweet tastes activate the brain's reward center; when the reward, in the form of calories, doesn't arrive, our brains send us out in search of more calories. So even if two people eat the same amount of food, the person who washes it down with a diet soda is more likely to eat additional calories in the coming hours. The other ways artificial sweeteners promote weight gain is by altering the microbiome, reducing satiety even further, and making us want to eat more.

- **Sugar damages cognition.** A diet high in sugar can damage the hippocampus, creating inflammation in the area of the brain that plays a crucial role in memory and learning. Sugary foods can also lower our levels of brain-derived neurotropic factor (BDNF), which is essentially human growth hormone for the brain; in an animal study, those put on a high-fat, high-sugar diet for two months showed reduced levels of BDNF and reduced learning ability.

    ◊ **But so do artificial sweeteners.** Studies indicate that artificial sweeteners can pass through the blood-brain barrier and accumulate in brain tissue. In one study, people who drank diet sodas for forty weeks showed abnormalities in their hippocampus and dysregulation of proteins involved in the growth and survival of brain cells.

- **Sugar causes pain.** Psoriasis, IBD, and rheumatoid arthritis are just some of the deeply uncomfortable conditions that sugar has been shown to make worse. A study in *Pain Reports* looked at 4,123 people with spine issues and found that consuming added sugars was associated with a 49 percent increased risk of chronic spinal pain; those who consumed more Power Plants—specifically fruits and whole grains—and more dairy reduced their risk of chronic pain by up to 26 percent.

    ◊ **But so do artificial sweeteners.** Increased inflammation means increased pain. One review of studies found that artificial sweeteners can negatively impact those with chronic inflammatory conditions like irritable bowel syndrome (IBS) and arthritis.

Extra-Delicious Special Section

30 Plants in Just 5 Smoothies

It's hard to overstate the importance of starting each morning with a punch of protein.

A study in the *Journal of Dairy Science* compared two groups of people: One group ate 12.4 grams of protein for breakfast, while the second ate a breakfast boosted with whey protein powder, resulting in a protein intake of 28 grams. Researchers found that those who ate the extra protein in the morning had lower blood sugar levels and reduced levels of appetite later in the day. Another study found that a high-protein breakfast will cut sensations of hunger 51 percent more than a low-protein breakfast. And research consistently shows that 25 to 30 grams of protein in the morning is crucial for helping us retain lean muscle mass as we get older.

And the fastest, easiest, most effective way to make your breakfast protein-packed is with a whey protein smoothie. (Whey has also been shown to be the most microbe-friendly form of protein available.)

Smoothies offer a unique opportunity not only to secure our muscular function and keep hunger at bay, but to maximize our plant intake as well. Indeed, you could hit your thirty plants in just five days by making these push-button smoothie recipes.

Like pizza, smoothies taste great no matter what you throw at them. (Although I'd think twice about a pepperoni and onion smoothie.) These recipes are just guidelines; you can mix and match, add and delete, ingredients at will.

Some smoothie basics:

- Add fluids first. This will help the blender in its quest to mash up everything evenly.
- Head in the freezer section direction. Frozen fruits are usually cheaper, and often more nutritious, than the fresh versions,

and they're available all year 'round. If you choose to use fresh, toss a handful of ice cubes into the blender alongside the rest of the ingredients.

- Freeze some bananas, which provide a terrific addition to almost any smoothie recipe. Pro tip: Peel them before you freeze them, otherwise the peels turn into little Kevlar vests that won't come off.
- Keep hemp seeds and flaxseeds in your pantry. When added to a smoothie, they practically disappear, taste-wise. But they are rich in omega-3 fatty acids and protein.
- Remember, juices don't count as Power Plants. While I've used a couple of juices in these recipes, I haven't counted them as part of your thirty.
- It's never a good idea to isolate, unless you're buying whey protein. "Whey isolate" has had the lactose removed, while "whey concentrate" still contains lactose—a lot of it. If you have even the slightest reactivity to lactose, or to dairy in general, choose the isolate. The guy sitting next to you on the bus will thank you.
- Vegan? Use a vegan protein powder instead of whey, but make sure it's a "complete" protein made from a variety of different plants, and look especially for the amino acid leucine, which is found in dairy but often hard to get from plant sources.

Oh No, I Made Too Much Smoothie!

Not a problem—you can store leftover smoothies in a couple of simple ways:

- Pour into a mason jar or other airtight container. "Airtight" is crucial here, as a smoothie left open to the environment of your fridge will not only absorb odors from your leftover garlic chicken stir-fry but will also begin to forfeit nutrients.
- Freeze it. Fill an ice cube tray with your leftover smoothie and store in the freezer. Breakfast just got easier: All you need to do is let the frozen chunks soften a bit, consume what you want, and then pop the rest right back into the freezer for a fast return to form.

Jolted Awake

If, like me, you live with a severe caffeine addiction (and, like me, have zero interest in breaking it), this smoothie will amp you up to face the day with the nutrition you need and the caffeine you crave.

INGREDIENTS

¾ cup iced coffee

Splash of whole dairy, soy, or oat milk (optional)

½ frozen banana

1 tablespoon peanut butter

1 tablespoon hemp seeds

¼ cup unsweetened whole wheat cereal (such as All-Bran or Trader Joe's)

½ tablespoon 100% cacao powder

¼ cup pine nuts

1 scoop chocolate whey protein

1–2 ice cubes (optional)

Daiquiris for Breakfast

What is that whispering sound coming from your blender? It's saying, "Add rum . . ." But try not to do that—unless you're serving this smoothie for dessert.

INGREDIENTS

Splash of orange juice

Squeeze of lime juice

½ cup plain Greek yogurt

½ frozen banana

¼ cup frozen coconut chunks

¼ cup frozen peach chunks

¼ cup frozen pineapple chunks

½ fresh mandarin orange, peeled

¼ **cup frozen mango chunks**
¼ **cup frozen raspberries**
1 scoop vanilla whey protein

Berry Nice!

The sweetness of the berries balances with the acidity of the grapefruit and pomegranate to create a mix of flavors that shows Mother Nature at her very brightest.

INGREDIENTS

¾ **cup almond or soy milk**
½ **grapefruit, peeled and seeds removed**
½ **cup frozen blackberries**
½ **pear, cored**
½ **cup frozen blueberries**
½ **cup pomegranate arils**
1 tablespoon almond butter
1 scoop vanilla whey protein

Kale to the Chief

This smoothie looks challenging at first—kale? parsley? oats?—but trust me, it blends up into the smoothest green machine you'll ever drink. The single date is enough to give the drink a lively sweetness.

INGREDIENTS

1 cup oat milk
½ **cup kale leaves**
½ **cup parsley**
¼ **cup cooked whole oats**
½ **tablespoon ground flaxseeds**
1 whole pitted date

1 scoop vanilla whey protein
2–3 ice cubes
Top with ¼ cup chia seeds.

My Cherry Amour

Can this smoothie help you find love? Maybe not, but it could help seal the deal the morning after . . .

INGREDIENTS

1 cup almond or soy milk
½ cup frozen pitted cherries
¼ cup frozen strawberries
¼ cup frozen cranberries
¼ cup unsalted cashews
½ cup baby spinach leaves
¼ ripe avocado, peeled and pitted
Pinch of cinnamon
Drop or two of vanilla extract
1 scoop chocolate whey protein

30 Plants in Just 5 Salads

Every meal and every snack should be an opportunity to seek out a new plant or two. Whether it's pizza or burgers, a plate of spaghetti or a burrito, just about every common food can be amped up with a few smart additions, whether it's some avocado slices and grilled onions nestled under your burger bun or a mix of black, red, and navy beans rolled into your tortilla.

But what if you wanted to guarantee that you'll hit your thirty plants automatically, every week, without having to think? What if you just wanted to make sure you got six new plants every single day for five days, and never had to worry about another meal?

Well, I've got you covered. All you need to do is whip up a different one of these salads every day for lunch or dinner, and pair it with the protein of your choice. (I've recommended some options, but the ultimate combo is up to you.) Follow the directions in these recipes, and you'll have your thirty different plants in no time.

The Spinach and Strawberry

It screams out springtime, but this combo will work for you year-round.

INGREDIENTS

> **2 cups fresh spinach leaves**
> **2 cups baby green lettuce leaves**
> **½ cup strawberries, sliced**
> **½ cup blood orange segments**
> **¼ cup picked tarragon leaves**
> **¼ cup almonds, sliced**

DIRECTIONS

Combine all ingredients in a large salad bowl.

TOP WITH

> **BLOOD ORANGE VINAIGRETTE**
> **¼ cup white wine vinegar**
> **¼ cup blood orange juice**
> **1 teaspoon Dijon mustard**
> **1 cup extra-virgin olive oil**
> **Salt + black pepper to taste**

SERVE WITH

Grilled chicken

Don't Go Chasing Watermelons

Crunchy, summery, and bright, this salad enlivens watermelon with just a hint of hotness and mint.

INGREDIENTS

- 3 cups seedless watermelon, peeled and diced
- 2 cups fennel (lightly salted to remove excess water), thinly sliced
- 1 cup jicama, peeled and diced
- ¼ cup jalapeño (seeds removed), finely diced
- ¼ cup picked mint leaves
- ¼ cup macadamia nuts (pistachios would be great, too!), crushed

DIRECTIONS

Combine all ingredients in a large salad bowl.

TOP WITH

CHAMPAGNE VINAIGRETTE
- ¼ cup champagne vinegar
- 1 teaspoon Dijon mustard
- 1 tablespoon honey
- 1 cup extra-virgin olive oil
- Salt + pepper to taste

SERVE WITH

Grilled shrimp

How Do I Get Rid of All These Tomatoes?

It's a common problem in August and September, as neighbors are constantly foisting their overabundance of red orbs on one another. Here's what to do with the bounty.

INGREDIENTS

> 2 cups fresh heirloom tomatoes (or whatever you have), cored and diced
>
> 1 cup English cucumbers, peeled, halved lengthwise, and cut in semicircles
>
> 1 cup honeydew melon, peeled and diced
>
> ½ cup pomegranate arils
>
> ¼ cup basil leaves (whole for presentation or thinly sliced)
>
> ¼ cup toasted walnuts, crushed

DIRECTIONS

Combine all ingredients in a large salad bowl.

TOP WITH

> **LEMON VINAIGRETTE**
> ¼ cup fresh lemon juice
> 1 cup extra-virgin olive oil
> Salt + black pepper to taste

SERVE WITH

Grilled salmon (bonus points if you use some basil pesto on that salmon)

The Butternut Beet

This cozy autumnal salad takes advantage of seasonal items like butternut squash, pumpkin seeds, and kale. Serve warm or at room temperature.

INGREDIENTS

1 cup fresh beets, scrubbed, trimmed, and diced
1 cup butternut squash, peeled and diced
4 cups baby kale leaves
1 small shallot, peeled and thinly sliced into rings
¼ cup toasted pepitas (pumpkin seeds)
¼ cup chives, thinly sliced

DIRECTIONS

1. Preheat the oven to 325°F.
2. Spray a roasting pan with a light coating of olive oil, and add beets and squash. Roast until tender, about 30 minutes.
3. Once they are cooled, combine beets and squash with all other ingredients.

TOP WITH

BALSAMIC VINAIGRETTE
¼ cup balsamic vinegar
1 teaspoon whole grain mustard
1 teaspoon oregano (optional)
1 cup extra-virgin olive oil
Salt + black pepper to taste

SERVE WITH

Grilled skirt steak

The Roast of Brussels

Unlike revenge, this is a dish best served warm. A perfect salad for when winter has finally set in.

INGREDIENTS

> 3 cups brussels sprouts, trimmed and halved
> 1 cup radicchio, cored and cut into large chunks
> ½ cup Granny Smith apples, cored and diced
> ½ cup dried cherries
> ½ cup scallions (greens and whites), thinly sliced into rings
> ½ cup toasted, salted peanuts, crushed

DIRECTIONS

1. Preheat the oven to 400°F.
2. Spray a roasting pan with a light coating of olive oil, and add brussels sprouts. Roast until charred, about 30 minutes.
3. Immediately add the brussels sprouts to a large salad bowl with the rest of the ingredients.

TOP WITH

> **APPLE CIDER VINAIGRETTE**
> ¼ cup apple cider vinegar
> ¼ cup maple syrup
> 1 tablespoon whole grain mustard
> 1 cup extra-virgin olive oil
> Salt + black pepper to taste

SERVE WITH

Grilled pork tenderloin

3

The 7-Day Challenge, and Why We Need It Now

A weeklong dietary scavenger hunt that will change the way you eat, feel, and live— forever.

Staying focused is hard.

I know, because right after I typed those four words, I looked over at my smartphone to see if anything interesting had happened in the ensuing three seconds. (Hey, what if Pete Davidson has a new girlfriend and I'm the last to know?)

We don't live in a time when patience, long-term thinking, and devotion to a goal are particularly well rewarded. We get derailed every moment of every day by a digital attention-control industry that is programmed to ping the reward center in our brain over and over and over again.

Fortunately, the Full-Body Fat Fix is designed to deliver an immediate impact on your health, your weight, and your mood, in less time than it takes to get over a bad cold.

In fact, the best way to think about the next seven days isn't as a nutrition program. It's more like a game—a scavenger hunt, actually. Your goal is to find, hidden in your fridge, your pantry, your garden, or the supermarket shelves, thirty different plants.

Write down what they are.

And then put them in your mouth.

JUMP-START YOUR WEIGHT LOSS

While there are some simple rules to this program, you'll find that it's actually pretty freeform. Only the first seven days could reasonably be considered "mildly challenging." Yet the results you're going to achieve in that limited time will be eye-opening.

Here's your assignment for the next seven days:

- **Start each day with a protein smoothie**, preferably incorporating whey protein.
- **Eliminate all refined carbs and sweets.** (Relax, it's seven days! You can go without a cookie for seven days, right? Next week you get to eat dessert again—in fact, it's part of the program!)
- **Limit whole grains to one serving per day.** That means whole grain bread, oatmeal, brown rice, corn, plus more exotic grains like quinoa, buckwheat, barley, and so on. Remember, try to vary these as much as possible: Whole wheat pasta one day, oat bran the next, corn on the cob the day after. (Each unique whole grain counts as a Power Plant, so don't forget to add it to your total!)
- **Eat thirty different whole plants.** List your plants using the 7-Day Challenge Tracking Log on page 75, or just write 'em down on the kitchen message board or on your phone's notes app. What matters is to seek out new and interesting plants that help you expand your palate—and to have fun doing it. (Remember, you only get to count each plant once. Enjoy your kale, kohlrabi, or kalamata olives, and then move on.)
- **Exercise three times**—a combination of aerobic and resistance training, selected from the simple mix-and-match workout plan starting on page 168. Research has actually identified what might be the single best possible workout for your microbiome. Simply pick three upper-body exercises, three lower-body exercises, and one core exercise, and add in a short aerobic workout. (You can split the aerobic and resistance training into two sepa-

rate workouts if you prefer, or knock it all out at once.) You can do this program in a gym with exercise machines or free weights, or at home with barely any equipment at all—I've given you the complete instructions on how to do it all.

Many diet programs come with phases, in which you eliminate certain foods, or eat massive quantities of certain foods, or only eat between the hours of 4 and 6 P.M. during full moons. For the most part, these phases are nothing but gimmicks.

The 7-Day Challenge isn't a gimmick. It's a fast-acting jump start that brings together the most powerful, most scientifically proven tools we have for successful short- and long-term weight loss. Over the next seven days, you're going to:

1. Jump-start rapid weight loss. By cutting out simple carbs like desserts and limiting whole grains to no more than one serving per day, you'll dramatically reduce the number of carbohydrates you're consuming for the first seven days. You'll still be eating the healthiest sources of carbs, in the form of fruits, vegetables, and legumes; you'll just be eating less than you might typically eat.

This powerful change to your diet is going to lead to sudden, rapid weight loss within the first week of this program, as much as five pounds in the next seven days. Is it magic?

Nope, it's a trick.

Here's how it works: Carbohydrates that aren't burned off right away are stored in the body as glycogen. But to store glycogen, the body needs water—every gram of glycogen stored in our bodies comes with three grams of water. When we reduce carbs, we start to burn off that glycogen—and shed the water weight.

That means you'll quickly notice a difference on the scale and in the way your clothes fit. And numerous studies have shown that rapid initial weight loss is predictive of long-term success. Essentially, if you see fast results, you're more likely to stick with the program over the long haul. So, one effect of the 7-Day Challenge is to demonstrate short-term success. And by doing that, you're essentially tricking yourself into long-term success.

You sneaky devil.

2. Enjoy tastes and flavors you've never experienced before. It's going to be fun to fill out your 7-Day Challenge Tracking Log, aiming to hit thirty different plants in a single week. You're going to love doing it this week. You might even want to do it again in weeks two or three. But eventually, you're going to get distracted and stop filling out your scorecard.

And that's fine.

By being mindful of maximizing your plant diversity in the first week, you're going to be discovering some new foods, trying out some new recipes, and breaking free of some of the conventions and habits that have guided the way you eat. Remember, even "healthy" eating habits become less healthy if we don't build diversity into our diets. Your goal over the next seven days is simply to break out of your current eating habits and find new foods that are going to enrich your life, foods you can incorporate into your meals in the months and years to come.

3. Stop and reverse muscle loss. Starting at around age thirty, we begin to lose about 5 to 6 percent of our total skeletal muscle every decade. For an idea of what this means, bend your arm and make a muscle. That bicep you're flexing is about 5 to 6 percent of your overall skeletal muscle. That means, by age fifty, the average person has lost two armfuls of muscle!

There's a simple reason why this happens: Our bodies are constantly breaking down and building up muscle tissue. But as we move past age thirty, the rate at which we break muscle down begins to exceed the pace at which we can rebuild it. The reason: a phenomenon known as *anabolic resistance*. Essentially, our bodies begin to have trouble turning the protein we eat into muscle, a problem that starts in our fourth decade and accelerates as we get older. To overcome this issue—to break through the resistance and ensure that we're not losing valuable, fat-fighting muscle—we need to eat larger doses of protein throughout the day. And while the average American eats an adequate amount of daily protein, we usually eat the majority of it at night. In fact, the typical American breakfast contains just 10 grams of protein, while the typical dinner contains 60 grams.

The single best thing you can do to stop, and reverse, age-related muscle loss is to start your day with protein. By mid-life, "A woman needs 25 grams of protein in the morning, and a man 30 grams," Jamie Baum, PhD, director of the Center for Human Nutrition at the University of Arkansas, told me. "Studies show that if you don't you could stay in muscle breakdown all day."

But getting 25 to 30 grams of protein at breakfast can be hard. A three-egg omelet contains just 18 grams of protein. A glass of milk, just 8 grams. And a 4-ounce container of fruit-on-the-bottom yogurt can have as little as 4 grams of protein (while being loaded with added sugars). That's why jump-starting your day with a protein smoothie is like taking out a free insurance policy on your muscles; it's a no-brainer way to ensure that you're getting the protein your body needs early in the day.

What about lunch and dinner? Chances are, you're probably already eating enough protein at lunch and dinner. But you can find suggestions for two weeks' worth of perfect lunches and dinners on page 215.

4. Completely remake your gut microbiome. Yes, in one week. One hundred trillion is a big number. If you've ever tried to get three cranky toddlers into a minivan, you know that being outnumbered in any way can make orderly transitions pretty impossible. So, the idea of getting 100 trillion microbes to all shift in one direction seems epic.

And yet science shows us that just one week is all you need to execute a painlessly simple regime change within your belly—to bolster diversity, tamp down the overpopulation of inflammatory microbes, and allow healthy new populations to gain purchase.

Our microbiome adapts to better manage the food that we feed it. And it does so quickly: In one study, young adults ate a plant-based diet consisting of fruits and vegetables, legumes, and whole grains for five days. After that, they returned to their normal diets. Then they were switched to an animal protein–based diet with lots of cheese, meat, and eggs for another five days. In each instance, the volunteers' microbiomes became wildly different after less than a week of following the different diets. Another study switched people to a Mediterranean diet for just three days and documented "immediate" and "reversible" changes to their microbiomes.

The 7-Day Challenge is just the first step (okay, the first seven steps) on this journey. But the jump start it gives you will power you forward and lay the foundation of a very simple eating plan that will serve you well for life.

SEE RESULTS . . . *WHEY* FASTER

This plan asks you to start each of your first seven days with a protein smoothie, preferably one made from whey protein. (Vegans and those with a true allergy to dairy can substitute plant-based protein powders.)

But . . . what even *is* whey? And why this type of protein versus any of the many other options out there?

If the only thing you know about whey is that Little Miss Muffet ate it, you're missing out on an incredibly powerful weapon in your battle to fight inflammation, retain lean muscle, stop fat gain, and heal your gut.

Until recently, whey was the overlooked side product of cheese-making, the leftovers discarded in the manufacturing process. About 80 percent of milk is casein, which is what is used to form your sharp cheddars, your smoked goudas, your triple-cream Bries, your fancy Pecorino Romanos. The other 20 percent is whey, and, for most of human history, whey has been used for little more than a) making ricotta, or b) slopping the hogs.

If casein is Beyoncé, whey is Solange.

But lately the overlooked sibling has been getting a lot more attention. While it's been a favorite of athletes and bodybuilders for years, more and more research is suggesting that we should all try to make it a regular part of our day. Among its superpowers, whey can:

- **Stop hunger—and keep it at bay.** Several studies have shown that whey protein has a stronger satiety effect than other proteins, including even whole milk, meaning it will keep you full and satisfied longer. That's primarily thanks to its high content of branch chain amino acids (BCAAs), crucial building blocks for muscle. One specific amino acid, leucine, reaches the brain rapidly after consumption, immediately signaling the appetite to switch off. In fact, leucine has been shown to control both short- and long-term appetite.

- **Build muscle—at any age.** Leucine seems to be almost a magic bullet for muscle gain; studies show that, particularly for people over forty, significant doses of leucine are critical for maintaining strength. But leucine is hard to find in substantial amounts in most foods other than animal proteins, and whey is far denser in leucine than just about any other food, including its sibling casein. That's why whey is such a potent muscle builder and fat fighter; as the late Doug Paddon-Jones, PhD, professor in the Department of Nutrition and Metabolism at the University of Texas Medical Branch, told me, "Whey protein is essentially a leucine delivery system that comes in chocolate."

- **Bring better health to your belly bugs.** Whey is an important component of breast milk and seems to play a significant role in helping infants develop a healthy microbiome and protect against the overgrowth of hazardous microbes like E. coli. And that salutary effect is duplicated each time we consume whey as adults. In one study, researchers tested the effects of whey protein supplements on the microbiomes of both normal weight and obese subjects. They found that the whey stimulated the growth of healthy probiotic bacteria and enhanced the production of SCFAs, while there was no growth of any family of bacteria associated with obesity. Researchers concluded that whey supplementation "may be an interesting approach to the prevention of overweight and obesity and related disorders." In a 2017 study of overweight people, those who ingested soy or casein protein supplements showed no change in their microbiota. But in a later study, this time in athletes, those who took whey supplements did show improvement in the number of healthy gut microbes. In addition, animal studies have shown that the quality of the protein being ingested makes a difference in the quality of the host's microbiome, and that whey seems to have a more beneficial effect than other types of protein.

- **Improve your mood and your sleep.** Whey is high in tryptophan, a precursor to serotonin, which helps to regulate not just mood but also appetite. (Antidepressants like Prozac work by boosting serotonin levels in the brain.) It helps improve our sleep and, as a result, our cognitive function, thanks to the serotonin-boosting effect.

- **Lower inflammation levels** by reducing pro-inflammatory enzymes, improving glucose management, boosting the health of blood vessels, and regulating adipokines, the hormones produced by your fatty tissue, including the appetite-squasher leptin.

Whey protein comes in two forms: concentrate and isolate. Whey concentrate is less expensive, but . . . whey isolate is the way to go if you have any sort of sensitivity at all to dairy. Whey isolate has had all of the lactose removed, which means even those who are lactose-intolerant and blow up at the mere idea of ice cream can safely use whey protein isolate.

The 7-Day Challenge Tracking Log

This extremely simple chart allows you to track your plant intake throughout the week, adding to your total of unique plants with every meal and snack. You'll see how you're doing on your quest to hit thirty, and be reminded to get creative to ensure you're feeding your microbiome all the nutrition it needs.

THE POWER PLANTS

VEGETABLES

- ☐ Artichoke
- ☐ Arugula
- ☐ Asparagus
- ☐ Beets
- ☐ Bell pepper (red, green, yellow, orange)
- ☐ Bok choy
- ☐ Broccoli
- ☐ Brussels sprouts
- ☐ Cabbage, green
- ☐ Cabbage, napa
- ☐ Cabbage, red
- ☐ Carrots
- ☐ Cauliflower
- ☐ Cucumber
- ☐ Eggplant
- ☐ Fennel
- ☐ Green beans
- ☐ Jicama
- ☐ Kale
- ☐ Leek
- ☐ Lettuce, Bibb
- ☐ Lettuce, green leaf
- ☐ Lettuce, red leaf
- ☐ Lettuce, romaine
- ☐ Mushrooms, portobello (also includes button and cremini—all the same plant)
- ☐ Mushrooms, shiitake
- ☐ Nori (sushi wrap)
- ☐ Onion
- ☐ Radish
- ☐ Scallion
- ☐ Snap or sweet peas

- ☐ Spinach
- ☐ Squash, summer
- ☐ String beans
- ☐ Tomato, beefsteak
- ☐ Tomato, cherry
- ☐ Tomato, grape
- ☐ Tomato, Roma
- ☐ Zucchini

FRUITS

- ☐ Acai
- ☐ Apple, Cortland
- ☐ Apple, Fuji
- ☐ Apple, Gala
- ☐ Apple, Granny Smith
- ☐ Apple, Red Delicious
- ☐ Apricot
- ☐ Banana
- ☐ Blackberries
- ☐ Blueberries
- ☐ Cantaloupe
- ☐ Cherries
- ☐ Cranberries
- ☐ Dates
- ☐ Figs
- ☐ Golden berries
- ☐ Grapefruit
- ☐ Grapes, green
- ☐ Grapes, purple
- ☐ Grapes, red
- ☐ Kiwi
- ☐ Mango
- ☐ Melon, casaba
- ☐ Melon, honeydew
- ☐ Mulberries
- ☐ Orange, blood
- ☐ Orange, mandarin
- ☐ Orange, navel
- ☐ Peach
- ☐ Pear, Asian
- ☐ Pear, Bartlett
- ☐ Pear, Bosc
- ☐ Pear, D'Anjou
- ☐ Pineapple
- ☐ Plum
- ☐ Pomegranate arils
- ☐ Raspberries
- ☐ Rhubarb
- ☐ Strawberries
- ☐ Tangerine
- ☐ Watermelon

STARCHY PLANTS

- ☐ Barley
- ☐ Beans, black
- ☐ Beans, kidney
- ☐ Beans, navy
- ☐ Beans, pinto
- ☐ Chickpeas and hummus
- ☐ Corn
- ☐ Lentils
- ☐ Oats
- ☐ Parsnip

- ☐ Peas
- ☐ Potato, red with skin
- ☐ Potato, sweet with skin
- ☐ Potato, white with skin
- ☐ Pumpkin
- ☐ Quinoa
- ☐ Rice, brown
- ☐ Rice, wild
- ☐ Squash, acorn
- ☐ Squash, butternut
- ☐ Turnip
- ☐ Wheat, whole grain

FATTY AND/OR PROTEIN-RICH PLANTS

- ☐ Almonds/almond butter
- ☐ Avocado
- ☐ Brazil nuts
- ☐ Cashews/cashew butter
- ☐ Chia seeds
- ☐ Coconut
- ☐ Flaxseeds
- ☐ Hazelnuts
- ☐ Hemp seeds
- ☐ Olives
- ☐ Peanuts/peanut butter
- ☐ Pecans
- ☐ Pine nuts
- ☐ Pistachios
- ☐ Pumpkin seeds (pepitas)
- ☐ Sesame seeds
- ☐ Soy (edamame, tofu, tempeh)
- ☐ Sunflower seeds/sunflower seed butter
- ☐ Walnuts

ADVENTURE CLUB!

The Power Plants already listed are common, but you might find yourself eating something interesting and altogether new: kohlrabi, dragon fruit, guava, or prickly pear.

Don't forget to write it down and give yourself credit for yet another Power Plant.

- ☐ _____
- ☐ _____
- ☐ _____
- ☐ _____
- ☐ _____
- ☐ _____
- ☐ _____
- ☐ _____
- ☐ _____
- ☐ _____
- ☐ _____
- ☐ _____
- ☐ _____
- ☐ _____

My Food Diary

7 Days to 30+ Plants

In case you have any doubts about how easy this program is—even the 7-Day Challenge!—take a look at my own personal journey through the first week.

MONDAY

Breakfast: Daiquiris for Breakfast whey protein smoothie (recipe, page 57) with banana, coconut, peach, pineapple, mandarin orange, mango, and raspberries.

Ideally, you'll start each day of the 7-Day Challenge with a whey-protein smoothie. In fact, if you follow each of the recipes on pages 55–66, you'll hit your thirty plants in just the first five days. But that requires a bit of shopping, so feel free to make up smoothies of your own, or just pick one or two recipes that best fit what you're craving. This recipe also includes orange juice and lime juice, but juices don't count, even if freshly squeezed. While the vitamins, minerals, and phytonutrients are retained in juice, the fiber is not, and it's fiber that's crucial for feeding the microbiome. I've used the juices here as a liquid base and flavor boost only.

Lunch: Panda Express String Bean Chicken, half order fried rice (brown rice, peas, carrots, and scallions), and "Super Greens" (kale, cabbage, and broccoli in light garlic sauce).

Panda Express packs eight different plants into this dish, which delivers 31 grams of protein and 10 grams of fiber.

Dinner: Chicken parmesan in homemade marinara sauce with mozzarella and parmesan cheese over chickpea pasta, and a side salad of romaine lettuce, pine nuts, balsamic dressing.

Pastas made with ingredients other than wheat are called "pulse" pastas; they can be made from an array of starches, such as lentils or rice, but chickpea pastas are packed with both protein and fiber and cook up to a consistency that's closest to real pasta. Also, I'd love to share our homemade marinara with you, but it has been passed down through my wife's family and she won't give me her recipe. Please consult your nearest Italian grandmother.

Unique Power Plants for the day: banana, coconut, peach, pineapple, mandarin orange, mango, raspberries, string beans, brown rice, peas, carrots, scallions, kale, green cabbage, broccoli, chickpeas, romaine lettuce, pine nuts. **Running total: 18.**

I'm off to an amazing start—more than halfway to thirty already, thanks to my plant-packed smoothie breakfast and well-ordered lunch.

TUESDAY

Breakfast: Berry Nice! whey protein smoothie (recipe, page 58) with fresh grapefruit, frozen blackberries, pear, frozen blueberries, pomegranate arils, almond butter, milk, and vanilla whey protein.

Frozen fruits can be as high (or higher) in nutrients as fresh fruits and are terrific choices for smoothies because they eliminate the need for extra ice.

Lunch: Slices of cheddar cheese and roasted turkey, side of coleslaw made from kale, green and red cabbage, brussels sprouts, shredded carrots, mayonnaise, salt, pepper, and celery seeds.

I might normally have had a turkey and cheddar sandwich, but during the 7-Day Challenge I'm having only one serving of (whole) grains per day, and I was looking forward to hamburgers tonight, so I skipped the bread. The slaw came from a prepackaged shredded mix that I combined with mayo and spices. (Celery seed and plenty of black pepper are key to a good slaw.) BTW: Amateur botanists know that red and green cabbages, kale, and brussels sprouts, as well as cauliflower, broccoli, bok choy, and kohlrabi, are all descendants of the same plant—Brassica oleracea, or wild mustard. But studies that have looked at dietary diversity haven't distinguished between different varieties, and the experts I've spoken to say that these foods are far enough apart to qualify as unique plants. The same goes for different varieties of apples, grapes, oranges, and so forth. The one exception is when plants are defined by their stage of ripeness: Green olives are just unripe black olives, and green bell peppers are just unripe red bell peppers. Portobello, button, and cremini mushrooms are all the same plant, just at different stages.

Dinner: Grilled hamburgers on whole wheat buns topped with avocado and blue cheese. Side salad of baby spinach, baby kale, sweet pea leaves, and baby bok choy.

This side salad sounds exotic, but it's just a mix I picked up in the grocery store.

Unique Power Plants for the day: grapefruit, pear, blueberries, blackberries, pomegranate, almonds, brussels sprouts, whole wheat, avocado, spinach, sweet peas, bok choy. Running total: 30.

I've hit thirty different plants, and it's only Tuesday! Mission (almost) accomplished! Let's see how high I can go . . .

WEDNESDAY

Breakfast: Daiquiris for Breakfast smoothie (recipe, page 57).

It's one of my favorites, and given that I'm already nearing my thirty-plant quota, I'll have it again.

Lunch: Chipotle Sofritas (crumbled tofu) Burrito Bowl with light cilantro-lime brown rice, black beans, fajita vegetables (bell peppers and red onion), tomato salsa, and Monterey Jack cheese.

While "sofritas" adds an additional plant to your day, this dish would still deliver five plants even if you chose an animal protein over the vegetarian option. As designed above, you're getting 27 grams of protein and 7.5 grams of fiber for lunch!

Dinner: Sneaky Salmon "Salad" (recipe, page 182) with artichoke hearts, kalamata olives, roasted red peppers, tomatoes, and herbs; and a side of roasted broccoli.

This salmon dish is a favorite even with my young daughter who hates anything that's not beige. To make perfect broccoli, lightly flash-boil it in a pot of water, transfer immediately to ice water, and drain thoroughly. Place on a baking pan, coat with olive oil and salt, and roast at 400°F for about half an hour.

Unique Power Plants for the day: soy (tofu), black beans, bell peppers, red onion, tomato, artichoke, kalamata olives. Running total: 37.

With seven unique Power Plants, I'm well beyond my thirty, and it's only Wednesday. What else does the week hold?

THURSDAY

Breakfast: Kale to the Chief whey protein smoothie (recipe, page 58) with kale, parsley, whole oats, flaxseeds, dates, chia seeds, and vanilla whey protein.

Since I'm only having one serving of (whole) grains per day, the oats in this recipe will count as my one serving. Fortunately, I get to eat more after the first seven days!

Lunch: Buffalo Wild Wings six-count traditional wings with signature sauce and carrots and celery with fat-free ranch.

Sometimes, getting in your plants is as simple as eating the colorful little sticks that come alongside your meal. In this case, I'm getting 32 grams of protein and 5 grams of fiber from this "decadent" lunch.

Dinner: The Spinach and Strawberry salad (recipe, page 62) with spinach, green baby lettuce, sliced strawberries, blood orange, tarragon leaves, and sliced almonds, served with grilled chicken.

These salad recipes are designed to get you to thirty plants in just five days; as with the smoothies, if you eat them all, you're a guaranteed winner!

Unique Power Plants for the day: parsley, oats, dates, celery, green lettuce, flaxseeds, chia seeds, strawberries, blood orange, tarragon leaves. Running total: 47.

FRIDAY

Breakfast: Berry Nice! whey protein smoothie (recipe, page 58).

Lunch: Waffle House Hashbrown Bowl with two eggs, grilled yellow onions, jalapeño peppers, Bert's chili (with pinto beans), grilled tomatoes, and grilled mushrooms.

This is a great example of how you can turn a classically "unhealthy" restaurant meal into a nutrition-packed meal. Order it "smothered" (with onions), "capped" (with mushrooms), "peppered" (with jalapeños), "diced" (with tomatoes), and "topped" (with chili). In addition to the base of potatoes, that's a lot of different plants!

Dinner: One-Skillet Coconut Curry Chicken Thighs and Vegetable Trio (recipe, page 204), with broccoli, summer squash, red bell pepper, whole wheat couscous, cashews, and cilantro.

Unique Power Plants for the day: potatoes, yellow onions, jalapeños, pinto beans, mushrooms, summer squash, cashews, cilantro. Running total: 55.

SATURDAY

Breakfast: My Cherry Amour whey protein smoothie (recipe, page 59) with frozen cherries, strawberries, cranberries, cashews, baby spinach, avocado, and chocolate whey protein.

Lunch: Spicy tuna roll from my local sushi joint, with brown rice and tuna wrapped in nori, plus edamame.

Don't forget that not every plant grows on land. Nori and other types of seaweed also count! Consider trying the seaweed salad the next time you order sushi—it usually comes with at least a couple of different types of seaweed, plus sesame seeds.

Dinner: Grilled steak with baked sweet potato fries and No More Sufferin' Succotash (recipe, page 185) with onion, red bell pepper, edamame, corn, asparagus, and bacon.

Unique Power Plants for the day: cherries, cranberries, nori, sweet potatoes, corn, asparagus. Running total: 61.

SUNDAY

Breakfast: Berry Nice! smoothie.

Lunch: Don't Go Chasing Watermelons salad (recipe, page 63), with seedless watermelon, sliced fennel, diced jicama, diced jalapeño, mint leaves, and crushed macadamia nuts, served with grilled shrimp.

Dinner: Pesto, Sausage, and Salad Flatbread Pizza (recipe, page 198) with basil pesto, whole wheat pita, mozzarella cheese, pistachios, turkey sausage, cherry tomatoes, and arugula.

During the 7-Day Challenge, I'm eating only whole grains—and this homemade pizza recipe uses whole grain pita. But in the coming weeks, I'll order pizzas from my local shop and have them load on veggies like artichoke, mushrooms, and onions.

Unique Power Plants for the day: watermelon, fennel, jicama, mint, macadamia nuts, pistachios, basil. Running total: 68.

WOW! I more than doubled my goal of thirty plants in a week, and I did it while eating pasta, pizza, steak, and hamburgers at home, and dining out at Buffalo Wild Wings, Panda Express, and Waffle House—none of which have ever been confused with "health food" restaurants.

Now *that's* an easy weight-loss plan to follow!

4

How the Full-Body Fat Fix Will Save Your Life (Over and Over Again)

From chronic discomforts to life-threatening conditions, your microbiome holds the key to battling the myriad diseases of aging.

Have you ever been told that to be healthier you need to lose weight? I hope the preceding chapters have convinced you to rethink that advice. Because, as we've seen, being overweight is not the *cause* of health issues like heart disease, diabetes, and arthritis. Instead, it's a parallel symptom. The same underlying issue of chronic inflammation that causes your fat cells to swell and immune cells to invade your fatty tissue is also the main driver of a vast majority of what we think of as the "diseases of aging."

In fact, in recent years experts have even coined a term for the myriad ways in which inflammation causes premature aging and, along the way, lays the table for everything from cancer to stroke to autoimmune disease: "inflammaging."

The great news, then, is that we don't have to worry about a lot of different diseases as we get older.

We just have to worry about one.

If we can keep inflammation down—by feeding and nurturing a healthy microbiome through a diverse, plant-based, protein-rich diet and moderate exercise—we can begin to make significant reductions in our risk of more than 100 different diseases, including top killers like cancer and heart disease, and less frightening but still extremely unfortunate issues like rheumatoid arthritis, celiac disease, psoriasis, Crohn's disease, Raynaud's disease, restless leg syndrome, ulcerative colitis, and endometriosis.

Look at all that you'll gain from following this program and the many ways it will make your life better for years to come.

GET A HANDLE ON HEART DISEASE

We all know that being obese increases our risk of heart disease. But why, exactly?

You might imagine that it's just a matter of mechanics: As we lug around more weight, our heart has to pump harder and push more blood. Well, that's true—but the same is true of elite athletes, bodybuilders, and the naturally ginormous. Nobody is looking at LeBron James or Dwayne Johnson and saying, "That guy's a walking heart attack."

It's not size that sets us up for heart attacks. It's the way our fat cells behave after the Big Bang we talked about in Chapter 1. It's the attack of inflammation.

As we've seen previously, one thing inflammation does is cause irritation to the various cells in your body. In your fatty tissue, irritated fat cells call out for help, causing macrophages to rush to the scene, which only causes more inflammation—as well as adding to the size of your belly.

Well, the same thing happens throughout your circulatory system. As microbial diversity declines and unhealthy bacteria take over, the lining of the gut becomes inflamed, allowing microbes and various toxic by-products from your gut to leak into the bloodstream. At the same time, that inflammation is causing your fat cells to fill to bursting, at which point fatty acids can also leak out into the bloodstream. These two factors cause irritation in the lining of your blood vessels, giving plaque a toehold—a condition known as atherosclerosis—and providing a starting point for blockages to form. Or that plaque can grow until it breaks off, traveling through your bloodstream until it becomes lodged in a vessel that services the heart. Either scenario can trigger a heart attack or, if the blockage happens in your brain, a stroke.

"Atherosclerosis is a chronic inflammatory disease," researchers wrote recently in the *International Journal of Molecular Disease*. (Remember how we read nearly the exact same sentence about obesity earlier in this book?) Much like your belly fat, the plaque in your arteries is made up of not just fatty substances but billions of immune cells that have been activated by—and continue to fan the flames of—inflammation. The immune cells in your bloodstream capture the cholesterol floating in your blood and bind it to your arteries, encapsulating it in solid chunks. Researchers have even shown that using a targeted anti-inflammatory called canakinumab lowers the rate of recurring cardiac events among patients who have suffered a heart attack. And most of the standard medical interventions for heart disease, including beta-blockers and statins, are anti-inflammatory in nature.

It's no coincidence, then, that all of the things that are considered good for your heart—plenty of fruits and vegetables, regular exercise, healthy fats, and stress reduction—are also good for your microbiome. Some foods increase inflammation, but you probably know what they are. They're the same foods everyone from your dentist to your cardiologist has warned you about. One study followed 2,735 men and women starting at age forty-nine. Over the ensuing thirteen years, women who ate the most sugary foods and the least amount of fiber were 2.9 times more likely to die from inflammation-based diseases such as heart disease.

PUT THE DAMPER ON DIABETES

As lipids and other toxins leak out into the bloodstream, putting us at risk for heart disease and stroke, they spread inflammation throughout the body. The lipids begin to accumulate in the liver and muscles, a condition known as "lipotoxicity," because these fatty acids are literally poison. The liver becomes inflamed and less effective at processing not only cholesterol but insulin as well, and becomes less efficient at storing excess blood sugar. The muscles become weaker, more "marbled," and, like the liver, they also become less effective at storing excess blood sugar.

Damage to these two crucial blood-sugar storage points means more sugar floating around in the bloodstream, which means the pancreas has to pump out more insulin to handle the influx. But inflammation also damages the body's insulin receptors, making us less efficient at turning that sugar into energy—a condition known as insulin resistance. With fewer places to store it and a reduced capacity for turning it into energy, the body has just one option: It directs all that excess sugar toward the fat cells in the belly, and they continue to swell, creating even more inflammation.

Macrophages continue to collect in the fatty tissue, responding but also contributing to the increase in inflammation. They secrete inflammatory substances that further interfere with insulin signaling and promote greater levels of insulin resistance. As more energy gets directed into the fat cells, they become stressed and die off; when they do, the macrophages gather around them, creating what's called "crown-like structures"— essentially inflammation haloes surrounding the dead fatty tissue.

Many of the most commonly prescribed diabetes treatments, such as metformin, have anti-inflammatory properties. And they have demonstrated just how powerful fighting inflammation can be. Indeed, several meta-analyses of studies have found that people who take metformin to treat diabetes live longer and suffer fewer of the diseases of aging (including heart disease, cancer, and cognitive decline) than the general population—even those who don't have diabetes!

BOOST YOUR RESISTANCE TO INFECTIOUS DISEASES

All of this toxicity coursing through your body keeps your immune system on high alert, the very definition of chronic inflammation. Your body is one million percent convinced that it's under attack. And it is, but from the inside.

Imagine an ambulance company that's never granted a moment of rest. All the EMTs are constantly racing around, gathering their gear, driving off to one emergency after another, only to discover false alarm after false alarm. The drain on the company's resources is tremendous: After a while, the ambulances start to run out of gas, the equipment starts to wear down, and the EMTs start to run out of enthusiasm. So, when yet another alarm goes off, they might not react as efficiently, or as effectively, as an ambulance with well-rested, well-stocked paramedics. That's a pretty good analogy for your immune system in the throes of chronic inflammation. Your body is so busy managing these ongoing, low-level crises that when a real emergency occurs it simply doesn't have the resources to respond as effectively as you might wish.

Researchers recently looked at how obesity and its silent partner, inflammation, affected outcomes for some 150,000 patients with COVID-19. Those with a body mass index (or BMI, a measure of body weight) of 30 to 34.9 (just above the "obesity" threshold) were 7 percent more likely to be hospitalized, and 8 percent more likely to die, than people who were a healthy weight. But as weight and inflammation increase, the risk increases as well: Those with a BMI of 45 or higher were 33 percent more likely to be hospitalized and 61 percent more likely to die. People with obesity are more likely to catch a severe case of the flu and more likely to die from it, too, and they often remain contagious for longer than healthy-weight folks.

As we've seen, inflammation also damages our ability to process leptin, the hormone that helps to control appetite—one of several sneaky ways that fat causes us to build more fat. But leptin also plays a role in the immune system, helping to regulate protective T cells—the first line of defense against a new invader. Studies show that as BMI increases, the number of T cells in the bloodstream decreases, hampering not just our ability to fight off infections but also to repair wounds. We become more likely to suffer skin infections, urinary tract infections, and advanced liver infections. We become more susceptible to bacterial, viral, and even fungal attacks.

And while our distracted immune system is failing to recognize these outside invaders, it can fail to recognize other threats as well.

Can This Device Help You Manage Your Microbiome?

What if you could have a top-notch diagnostician monitoring your body 24/7, picking up on health issues long before symptoms arose? And a fitness and nutrition coach who could tell you exactly how your body would react to your next meal, and the absolute best time to exercise to get maximum benefits? And what if that doctor-in-your-pocket could also continuously monitor your blood sugar, cholesterol, blood pressure, and even stress levels, and tell you precisely what to do in the coming hours to help keep it under control?

Sounds like something out of *Billions* or *Succession*, but you don't need to be a master of the universe to have a constant health coach by your side. Continuous glucose monitors (CGMs) are becoming more and more popular as a way of fully understanding how our bodies are reacting to the world around us. And while they were originally developed as a way of helping diabetics control their glucose levels without frequent finger pricks, more and more non-diabetics are using these devices off-label to gain insight into their health—and their microbiomes. Companies like Nutrisense, Levels, and January AI are using CGMs on people to detect larger health issues.

"When you go to the doctor, he or she will take a bunch of measurements, but those results will be measured against population averages—not your particular physiology," says Michael Snyder, PhD, director of the Center for Genomics and Personalized Medicine at Stanford University and cofounder of January AI. But a CGM can measure current you against healthy you—and instantly detect when something is wrong. An ongoing study of 109 people using January AI has, as of this writing, uncovered 49 different health issues among that cohort—including cancers and heart issues—before symptoms became apparent. Indeed, January AI was able to detect COVID-19 infections in users an average of four days before the onset of symptoms. (The device even detected that Snyder had Lyme disease before the onset of symptoms, he said.)

Snyder said that because each of us has a distinct microbiome, we each react to specific foods in different ways. By building a "model" of your body, January AI can identify which foods spike your glucose levels and which don't. It can also monitor the way that plant fibers interact with your microbiome. For example, we know that oatmeal supposedly lowers cholesterol. But how? "Everyone used to think that arabinoxylan [the type of fiber found in whole oats, as well as wheat, barley, and other grains] just directly binds with cholesterol," Snyder said. "But now we think that it promotes bacteria that metabolize cholesterol into bile acid."

What we're learning from these CGMs is that our unique microbiomes can be maximized by eating a wide variety of fibers and seeing how our bodies react. And that's particularly true for the estimated one in three of us who is prediabetic. (Not you? Don't be so sure—about 80 percent of people who are prediabetic don't know it, Snyder said.) While insulin is controlled by the pancreas, the hormones that stimulate insulin are produced by the epithelial cells in the colon. And that's the microbiome's playground.

PUT THE KIBOSH ON CANCER

As your immune system continues to pump out inflammatory compounds—attempting to fight fire with fire—it loses the ability to measure and respond to real dangers. It has trouble detecting unhealthy cells that are growing out of control, which is one reason why obesity is associated with cancers of the breast, uterus, ovary, esophagus, stomach, colon, liver, gallbladder, pancreas, kidney, thyroid, and others.

And a confused immune system is just one factor in the dramatic increase in cancer risk caused by out-of-control inflammation. One of the things our bodies do to combat tissue damage—which is exactly what's happening in your belly as fat cells swell and leak—is to produce reactive oxygen and nitrogen species (RONS), which you might know by the more common name "free radicals." These molecules help to repair and regenerate tissue, but they can also cause DNA damage, resulting in mutations that can promote cancer.

Our bodies are constantly breaking down, rebuilding, and duplicating our DNA. But as we age, our cells begin to have a more difficult time accurately repairing our DNA. Think of a copy machine that's running low on ink; the messages encoded in the document get harder and harder to read. Mistakes become duplicated, and so instead of the original, healthy roadmap set out for us at birth, we get a confusing set of instructions. A healthy microbiome helps to counteract this dilemma by creating metabolites—compounds like butyrate and others—that improve the body's ability to repair and correctly reproduce its own DNA. And by dampening inflammation, the microbiome can help prevent DNA damage in the first place.

Tackling inflammation is a promising field of study for cancer researchers. In one study, researchers testing the anti-inflammatory drug canakinumab—the same drug being researched as a treatment for heart disease—found that it reduced mortality from lung cancer by 77 percent.

TAKE ACTION AGAINST AUTOIMMUNE DISEASES

Let's go back to that ambulance company for a second: all those frantic paramedics—representing your immune system—running around in a chaotic state, trying to manage emergencies that in many cases don't exist. Yet the sirens are blaring, the ambulances are racing to and fro, and the paramedics are rushing around unhinged.

It's not hard to see how something's going to get broken here.

That's sort of what's happening inside your body when chronic inflammation rages, and it helps to explain one of the most unnerving phenomena of the past few decades—the dramatic rise in autoimmune disease.

You've probably heard a lot about autoimmune disease over the last decade, and for good reason. Celebrities like Selena Gomez and Kim Kardashian (both have lupus) and Venus Williams (Sjögren's syndrome, which causes dry eyes and joint pain) have gone public with their personal struggles, and autoimmune diseases played a role in the deaths of older stars like Eagles cofounder Glenn Frey and filmmaker and comedian Harold Ramis.

Autoimmune disease is caused when those chronically overtaxed EMTs become confused and start trying to do metaphorical chest compressions on otherwise healthy tissue. One theory for the rise of these diseases—which include rheumatoid arthritis, irritable bowel syndrome (IBS), multiple sclerosis, psoriasis, Hashimoto's disease, and type 1 diabetes—is that our microbiomes are becoming less diverse. As a result, inflammation rises, and autoimmune diseases become more common. At the same time, we're exposed to more and more chemicals—in our food, our drinking water, and our air—any of which may trigger inflammation in some people.

If you suffer from an autoimmune issue, you probably don't need convincing of the role that inflammation is playing in your health. All you need to do is look at how your body reacts to intense stress; it's not uncommon for people who have issues like psoriasis or IBS mostly under control to suffer flare-ups when stress hits. The reason: Under stress, our bodies release the hormone cortisol, which does a number of things that are very helpful in evading saber-toothed tigers and marauding hordes of Visigoths, but not so effective in meeting work deadlines or negotiating difficult social situations. Cortisol causes our blood pressure to spike, our heart rates to rise, our blood to clot more easily—and yes, it raises inflammation levels. These are all positive changes when you're anticipating the need to quickly heal any wounds resulting from tiger bites or Visigoth swords. But they're not very useful when the stress is caused by crotchety bosses, clamoring toddlers, or crunchy traffic patterns.

Chronic stress, by the way, has been shown to damage the microbiome. We'll look at some approaches for managing stress in Chapter 5.

GROW STRONG, NOT FRAIL

It's not in brittle bones, wasted muscles, or inflexible joints that frailty can first be spotted, but in the microbiome. In one study, researchers looked at the microbiomes of 728 sets of female twins between the ages of forty-two and eighty-six. They found that the less diverse a woman's microbiome, the higher she scored on a frailty index that measured things like an individual's need for help lifting objects, getting up and down stairs, or getting dressed.

Researchers analyzed gut microbiomes as well as other data from 9,000 people ages 18 to 101. They found that those whose microbiomes got more diverse with age were healthier and lived longer than their peers with less-diverse guts. They were able to walk faster, had lower levels of LDL (bad) cholesterol, higher levels of vitamin D, and higher levels of certain blood metabolites, created by gut microbes, that helped to reduce inflammation.

Oh, and one more benefit: Those with the most diversity in their microbiomes were also less likely to die during the course of the study.

Six Surprising Ways a Growing Belly Changes Your Body

In this chapter, we've talked exclusively about all the things that are happening inside your body as your belly grows and inflammation sets in. But while chaos is happening invisibly inside you, the larger effects are evident in the mirror. Belly fat does some pretty weird things to your physique:

Belly fat moves your ears. When you were younger, your ears were directly over your shoulders, exactly where they should be today. Indeed, when you stand erect, your ears, shoulders, hips, knees, and ankles should all be in alignment. This is the powerful posture we think of when we imagine a fit, healthy athlete striding out onto the playing field. But with age, you may notice that your ears are several inches out in front of your shoulders and that you're developing a bit of a hunch at the back of your neck. We typically blame this posture on too much time sitting at the desk, staring at the computer screen, but this "forward head" position became common long before Jobs, Gates, and Dell convinced us we needed computers in every home. It's caused by belly fat: As your belly grows outward, your center of gravity shifts; as a result, your body compensates by shifting your posture so you don't fall forward onto your chest.

Belly fat makes your butt stick out. As your abdomen spills forward, your pelvis tilts forward to accommodate the shift in weight, and your butt juts outward. This is called an anteriorly rotated pelvis. Your stomach muscles are being stretched and elongated, which weakens them, allowing more of your stomach to spill out. The hip flexors, which run down the side of your hip-bone and connect to your knee (you use them to lift your knee as if in a marching band), become shortened, while the hamstrings and butt muscles get pulled tight and stretched, weakening them as well.

Belly fat causes "rib flare." Yikes! What even is that? The combination of slouched shoulders, expanded belly, and tilted pelvis causes your chest to sink, which impedes on your diaphragm. Your body responds by pushing outward on your lower ribs, which is why the area right below your chest and under your arms also seems to expand. Normally, our torsos have a V shape, in which the top of the rib cage, just below the collarbone, is the widest part, and it tapers as it gets lower. But as fat accumulates, and posture deteriorates, the bottom of the rib cage expands, making us look heavier than we are.

Belly fat makes you walk funny. When it comes to our back, hips, and knees, many of the pains we feel don't have anything to do with our back, hips, and knees. As your belly spills out and your hips tilt forward, there's a pulling along the hamstrings, those big long muscles at the back of your thighs that connect to your lower back, as well as the iliotibial band (or ITB), a big band of connective tissue that runs down the outside of your thighs, connecting your hips to the sides of your knee. As the hamstrings and ITB get stretched, they pull on the lower back, the outsides of the hips, and various spots in the knee. "Bad knees," a "bad back," or "sore hips" may not indicate that there's anything wrong with any of these spots; it's simply that the pelvic tilt is creating tension and muscle imbalances that you're experiencing as physical pain. So you hobble along, not realizing that it's your belly that's making life so challenging.

Belly fat makes you shorter. It was once believed that carrying extra pounds was protective of bone mass. But recent research has shown that inflammatory visceral fat is associated with a greater risk of osteoporosis and bone fracture. The reason may have to do with the fact that those of us with the most visceral fat also have the most fat inside of our bones, in the marrow. (That's right—belly fat makes your bones get fat, from the inside.) Bone tissue is constantly breaking down and being rebuilt, but visceral fat interferes with the rebuilding process by reducing your body's levels of growth hormone (GH) as well as insulin-like growth factor 1 (IGF-1), a second hormone that regulates the body's use of growth hormone. As GH and IGF-1 drop, so does your body's ability to rebuild bone—as well as muscle. Eroding bone quality plays a main role in why people become shorter as they age, as vertebrae contract and connective tissues become weaker. Speaking of which:

Belly fat makes your muscles flabby. We call it "marbling," and it's great when you're selecting a choice ribeye, but it's less great when it happens to the muscles in your own body. More fat in the muscles means less strength and mobility. Indeed, the infiltration of fat into muscle tissue may explain why we lose strength with age even if we don't appear to lose muscle mass; simply put, the muscle isn't as high quality as it once was. In a study of older adults with a history of falls who began a resistance-training program, only those with low levels of intramuscular fat were able to significantly improve their muscle quality. Another study found that those with the most intramuscular fat were up to 80 percent more likely to develop mobility limitations over the following two and a half years, compared to those with the least marbling in their muscles. Researchers point to a direct line between inflammatory belly fat and inflammatory muscular fat; both send out cytokines that damage the tissue around them.

5

Listening in on the Conversation Between Your Belly and Your Brain

Want to become effortlessly happier and calmer while reducing your risk of cognitive decline? We know 100 trillion friends who can help.

Imagine going into a psychologist's office, reclining on a big leather chaise next to a conveniently placed box of tissues, and hearing the therapist ask that famous opening question:

"Tell me about your microbiome."

It might be a more effective—if less cathartic—approach toward changing your mindset than simply blaming everything on your parents. Indeed, researchers recently identified thirteen different species of gut microbes that may influence our risk of depression. In the study, researchers found that the differences in the guts of those with and without mood disorders were so striking that, simply by reading the makeup of an individual's microbiome, they could diagnose whether or not that person was depressed.

Did these bacteria withhold love at a crucial point in our childhoods? Did they smother us with overprotectiveness? No. But certain microbes play an important role in the synthesis of key brain-regulating chemicals that powerfully influence mood. And by determining the levels of inflammation in our bodies, our gut microbes help determine how well we sleep and how we react to stress; they play a role in our memory, our mood, and our cognitive function. The health of the microbiome, and its ability to metabolize our food properly, has been linked to everything from chronic fatigue syndrome to restless leg syndrome, from autism to schizophrenia, from Alzheimer's to alcoholism.

And that is opening an exciting new line of potential treatments for brain diseases. In a 2020 review, researchers looked at twenty-eight studies that involved a fecal microbiota transplant (FMT) between people who were psychiatrically ill and those who were not. In the studies, people who suffered from anxiety and depression saw a reduction in their symptoms after receiving transplants from healthy patients. But the inverse was also true: When healthy patients received FMTs from people who were depressed and anxious, the healthy individuals became depressed and anxious, too.

In other words, depression and anxiety can be contagious.

You get them from poop.

YOUR GUT DECIDES: WHETHER YOU'RE HAPPY OR SAD (OR ANXIOUS)

You've no doubt felt a butterfly garden in your gut when called on to speak in public, or maybe experienced a certain twisting queasiness when confronted with an unfortunate truth. Those "gut feelings" aren't just your mind playing tricks on you; they're a real phenomenon.

Our microbiome and our brain are in constant contact through the enteric nervous system (ENS)—a second brain, if you will, made up of specialized nerve cells located in the tissues of our digestive tract. The ENS sends signals to our main brain to tell us not just when we're hungry or when we're full but when we're feeling nauseous or nervous or neglected. More than 90 percent of the serotonin in our bodies—the very neurotransmitter that antidepressants are designed to boost—is produced in the gut by the ENS, which also plays a role in the creation of dopamine, the "reward" hormone that kicks in to make pleasurable sensations linger.

Those sensations, good and bad, originate with our microbiome. As our microbes munch on plant fibers, they produce short-chain fatty acids (SCFAs), compounds that activate certain receptors on the vagus nerve—the largest nerve in the body, one that reaches down from the brain and all the way into the intestinal tract. The vagus nerve modulates a wide array of physical and psychological processes, including digestion, inflammation, and mood. Oxytocin, the "love" hormone that inspires us to bond with others, is stimulated by the action of the microbiome on the vagus nerve. This giant nerve also plays a role in moderating our heart rate and breathing, as well as influencing the hormones that regulate digestion and appetite.

The vagus nerve is like a brake on our overall nervous system; the more activated it is, the calmer and more controlled we are. When the vagus nerve senses stress, however, it can become less active: Heart and breathing rates increase, and digestive activity slows—a part of the "fight or flight" response.

But a healthy gut microbiome can activate the vagus nerve and calm the stress response. In one French study, subjects were administered either probiotics (a mix of healthy microbes) or a placebo. Those who received the probiotics reported significantly reduced levels of psychological distress. In another study, healthy men and women who reported a depressed mood received probiotics or a placebo. Those who got the probiotics reported an improved mood over the course of the next three weeks (but those who received the placebo did not).

How is this possible? The driving force in depression, as with so many other diseases and disorders, is inflammation. Studies have shown that people who have been diagnosed with depression often have elevated levels of inflammatory markers in their blood and cerebrospinal fluid. In fact, one way that antidepressants work is by decreasing inflammation; studies of patients being treated for depression show that the higher one's inflammation levels at the beginning of treatment, the less likely that patient is to find relief. (Interestingly, talk therapy has also been shown to help lower inflammation.)

This helps explain why depression is more common among people with inflammatory diseases, from asthma and allergies to multiple sclerosis and lupus. Among people with diabetes, depression is twice as likely compared to those who don't have the disease.

A healthy microbiome impacts mood not only by reducing inflammation but also by downregulating the "fight or flight" response, and by generating and regulating mood-boosting neurotransmitters like serotonin. One study found that those whose guts were rich in a particular strain of gut bacteria showed higher levels of self-esteem. Other studies have shown that the health of our microbiomes might affect how popular we are, or how likely we are to fall in love.

The Meditative Microbiome

Researchers looking into the connection between mindfulness and the microbiome took stool and blood samples from thirty-seven Tibetan Buddhist monks who had been practicing meditation for an average of two hours a day for at least three years. For comparison, they also took samples from residents who lived near the monasteries and ate similar diets. They found, compared to the general population, the monks' microbiomes were more highly populated by specific bacteria that have been linked to lower levels of depression and anxiety, while their blood showed reduced levels of inflammatory markers linked to cardiovascular disease.

But you may not need to cloister yourself away for years to enjoy the benefits of meditation. In another study, forty-eight subjects with inflammatory bowel disease underwent nine weeks of mindfulness and relaxation-response training, participating in a weekly training session and practicing at home for fifteen to twenty minutes per day. They showed markedly decreased symptoms, as well as reduced anxiety and an improved quality of life.

YOUR GUT DECIDES: YOUR COGNITIVE FUNCTION AND ALZHEIMER'S RISK

There's no more frightening diagnosis than Alzheimer's disease; anyone who has watched a loved one slowly disappear before their eyes knows that dementia is a merciless thief. And yet, modern science—which has made such enormous strides in improving outcomes for people with diabetes, heart disease, cancer, and other diseases of aging—has proven remarkably inept at treating Alzheimer's.

Why? One reason might be our out-of-control levels of inflammation.

"There is an epidemic of diseases that are linked to inflammation," said Shilpa Ravella, MD, a gastroenterologist and assistant professor of medicine at Columbia University Medical Center, whose book on inflammation is titled *A Silent Fire: The Story of Inflammation, Diet & Disease*. "Obesity, high blood sugar, high blood pressure. We know that the blood-brain barrier is permeable, and that inflammation in the body can travel to the brain."

Increased permeability in the blood-brain barrier is a hallmark of Alzheimer's disease. One theory is that as cells in the brain become inflamed, they become less efficient at storing information, Ravella said. Hence, memory loss and the onset of dementia.

"The gut microbiome is a master controller of inflammation," said Sidhanth Chandra, researcher at Northwestern University Feinberg School of Medicine, who was the lead author on a recent paper examining the current state of research into the connection between Alzheimer's disease and the microbiome. "When you have long-standing inflammation, and long-standing changes in the microbiome, toxins from the bacteria in your gut are activating your immune cells both outside and inside of your brain," he told me. One current theory as to why people with Alzheimer's show a buildup of protein tangles in the brain is that these proteins, rather than being the cause of dementia, are simply the residual evidence. Normally, the immune cells in the brain, called the microglia, help to clear out these tangles. But when the microglia become exhausted from battling inflammation, they're simply not as good at getting rid of the debris, Chandra said.

Some research suggests that compounds generated by the gut microbiota may also travel to the brain via the vagus nerve, and that this pathway may further explain the connection between the gut and the brain. (There's even some evidence to suggest that the brain has a microbiome of its own, although researchers are still exploring this possibility.)

And in a groundbreaking 2023 study, researchers at the University of Pennsylvania found that the microbiome's influence over serotonin levels may be the cause of a confounding medical condition: long COVID, a syndrome defined by brain fog, depression, fatigue, and numerous other symptoms that linger for months or even years after the virus that causes COVID has been cleared from the bloodstream.

The researchers found that people with long COVID symptoms still had remnants of the virus in their guts, as well as reduced levels of serotonin. They speculated that the virus was interfering with the microbiome's ability to regulate serotonin, creating a situation in which sufferers were unable to retain new memories and otherwise shake off their post-COVID funk.

But regardless of how the bugs in your belly are communicating with your brain, we know that this conversation is continuous—and critical—and that the gut microbiomes of those with Alzheimer's are significantly different from those with healthy minds. One study looked at twenty-five people with Alzheimer's and twenty-five without; researchers found that those with the disease had gut microbiomes that were less diverse than those with healthy brains. Additional studies on the brain and the gut have reached the same conclusion: In a review of literature in the journal *Nutrition Reviews,* researchers found that "modulating the gut microbiome through specific nutritional interventions and the use of prebiotics and probiotics might represent an effective strategy to reduce the level of chronic inflammation and [amyloid proteins] associated with [Alzheimer's disease], possibly preventing or ameliorating [Alzheimer's] symptoms." And a meta-analysis of five studies involving nearly 300 patients, published in a 2020 edition of the journal *Aging,* found that probiotics improved cognitive performance in people with Alzheimer's or mild cognitive impairment, as well as lowering their levels of inflammation.

Unfortunately, the probiotics used in scientific studies such as these differ dramatically from what you might buy over the counter at your local Walgreens. Scientific studies typically use specific strains of bacteria in much higher dosages and much more tightly controlled quality than what's available at retail. That's why our diet is so important when it comes to healing the microbiome, fighting inflammation, and warding off cognitive decline, Ravella told me.

"When you take a probiotic pill, you're getting a few different strains of bacteria," she explained. (In fact, over-the-counter probiotics are, for regulatory reasons, limited to just three common strains.) "But when you eat a probiotic food [such as yogurt or sauerkraut], you have a wide range of bacteria that have developed together.

"Just as important for brain health is the diversity of your diet," Ravella said, adding that she currently lives in Hawaii in part because its vast natural resources—from its many opportunities to enjoy the outdoors to its wide array of exotic fruits and vegetables—offer a particularly healthy lifestyle for the microbiome. "The fruit here in Hawaii is amazing. Papaya just falls off the trees, and we have these little bananas called apple bananas, as well as mountain apples and star fruit."

Increasing the array and volume of whole foods in your diet has been shown to be a strong defense against cognitive decline. Adults fifty and younger who consumed 20 percent of their calories from ultra-processed foods showed a 28 percent faster rate of cognitive decline and a 25 percent faster rate of executive function decline compared to those who ate lower amounts, according to a 2022 study in *JAMA Neurology*. Another study published the same year looked at 1,070 adults aged sixty and older and found that those who ate the most fiber-rich foods showed greater cognitive function than those who ate the least.

Researchers are now looking for ways to improve brain health using this connection between fiber, the microbiome, and the mind. In one study, 818 people diagnosed with Alzheimer's were treated with either a placebo or a finely tuned prebiotic called GV-971 (a mix of plant fibers designed specifically to feed and encourage the growth of brain-healthy microbes). Those who received the prebiotic showed significant and sustained improvements in cognition over the course of the thirty-six-week trial, as well as reduced levels of inflammation in the brain.

Scientists are also able to consistently show progress in treating the disease in animal studies. When mice with an Alzheimer's-related mutation were treated with probiotics, they showed improved performance on recognition tests, reduced brain damage, decreased plaque buildup in the brain, and reduced inflammation. In another study of mice bred to develop Alzheimer's, those that received high-fiber prebiotics showed not only a healthier gut microbiome but also decreased cognitive defects and increased activation of immune cells in the brain.

Fecal microbiota transplants may also offer a future path to treating brain disease by improving the microbiome. When mice with Alzheimer's were given transplants from healthy mice, they showed reduced evidence of disease-related brain damage and improved performance on cognition tests.

That being said, the field of study linking the gut microbiome to Alzheimer's and other brain disease is "still in its early stages," Richard Isaacson, MD, director of the Florida Atlantic University Center for Brain Health, told me recently. But he has already seen a significant and demonstrable correlation between the health of the oral microbiome and brain inflammation.

"We've started focusing on tracking people's oral microbiome, identifying people with inflammatory markers in their bloodwork who also have other risk factors [for brain disease]," he said. "We had a patient who had persistent inflammation in his bloodwork, and we sent him to a specialist in oral health." The patient showed considerable periodontal problems—bleeding gums, gaps between his teeth and gums, and poor oral hygiene. After treatment, "within six months all his inflammation went down, even his cholesterol went down," Isaacson marveled. "So we have direct evidence that the oral microbiome, for one, can directly impact inflammation" and hence determine risk for Alzheimer's and other brain health issues.

Recent research has also linked the microbiome to the onset of Parkinson's disease. Researchers at the University of Alabama at Birmingham have found that two microbes, Lactobacillus and Bifidobacterium, are both overrepresented in the guts of people with Parkinson's. And here's another reason why trying to rebalance your microbiome with pills isn't a good idea: These are also the microbes that tend to be most common in over-the-counter probiotics.

YOUR GUT DECIDES: HOW YOU'RE GOING TO SLEEP TONIGHT

One of the biggest identifiable risks for Alzheimer's is impaired sleep: People with the disease often display disrupted sleep and dysregulated internal clocks, and those who struggle to sleep in mid-life are more likely to develop the disease in the future.

And the quality of your sleep is determined, in large part, by the bugs in your belly.

When you first lie down at night, your microbiome triggers the immune cells in your intestines to produce a variety of compounds that induce non-REM sleep—the deep, healing sleep that comes at the beginning of the night. (Cortisol, the stress hormone, inhibits the immune system from synthesizing these compounds, which is why we have trouble falling asleep when we're anxious.)

But when the microbiome becomes dysfunctional, it can produce higher levels of these compounds, which has the opposite effect: They not only prevent us from falling asleep at the beginning of the night but also increase our levels of depression and anxiety; impair long-term memory; and boost our sensitivity to pain. And that begins a cycle of poor sleep that further disrupts the microbiome: Researchers writing in the journal *Gut Microbes* found that long-term sleep disruption may indirectly lead to an unbalanced microbiome by altering eating and lifestyle habits, hence setting us on the path to Alzheimer's.

Poor sleep increases inflammation in the body, but a healthy microbiome may help to overcome that; several studies have shown that treating sleep patients with probiotic or prebiotic supplements improves REM and non-REM sleep.

YOUR GUT DECIDES: WHETHER TO HAVE THAT SECOND (OR FIFTH) DRINK

As researchers study the brain seeking to understand why some people become alcoholic and others don't, they've begun to key in on an unexpected explanation for alcohol addiction and withdrawal: the microbiome.

Since the 1980s, researchers have known that the intestinal fluid taken from alcoholics more commonly contains unhealthy bacteria such as E. coli or salmonella compared to their nonalcoholic peers. In 2014, researchers found that alterations in the microbiome among alcoholics, and the resulting decrease in intestinal barrier integrity—that is, leaky gut—can lead to depression, anxiety, and alcohol craving. People with alcohol use disorder produce less kynurenic acid (KYNA), a compound that's created in the liver, kidneys, and intestines and helps to protect the brain and nervous system. Lower blood plasma levels of KYNA and other protective compounds are correlated with alcohol cravings and depression; they're also associated with an increase in certain unhealthy gut bacteria. Even among alcoholics, the level of gut microbe dysfunction and leaky gut syndrome correlates with the degree of alcohol cravings, depression, and anxiety; when researchers divided chronic alcoholics into groups with greater or lesser levels of leaky gut and kept them free of alcohol consumption for three weeks, those with the greater degree of intestinal permeability also showed the greater degree of depression, anxiety, and alcohol cravings. This group also showed the lowest levels of specific healthy, anti-inflammatory microbes.

In a small 2021 study of twenty men with alcohol use disorder and cirrhosis, researchers gave half the subjects fecal microbiota transplants from healthy individuals; the other half received placebos. Among those who received the new microbes, 90 percent reported reduced alcohol cravings (versus 30 percent of the control group) at the six-month mark. The men also showed improved microbial diversity, lower levels of inflammatory compounds, improvements in cognitive function, and improved social interactions.

Of course, the link between alcoholism and gut microbes is a tough one to pin down. Does chronic alcohol abuse—and the generally unhealthy diet and other lifestyle factors that come with it—lead to a damaged microbiome? Or does the makeup of our microbes make some of us more susceptible to becoming alcoholic? Researchers writing in the *Journal of Medicinal Food* theorize that in about a third to a half of all alcoholics, it's the booze consumption that alters the gut microbiome, depleting protective species, increasing leaky gut, and sparking inflammation.

YOUR GUT DECIDES: WHETHER YOU'RE SOCIALLY ACTIVE OR LONELY

Like Alzheimer's, insomnia, and depression, loneliness can be considered an inflammatory condition.

In a study of 222 older adults, researchers found that those who scored higher on two different measures of loneliness also had higher levels of the inflammatory marker C-reactive protein in their blood, while another study of people aged eighteen to ninety-two found the same thing—being isolated or feeling lonely was linked to higher levels of inflammation.

Part of this has to do with the fact that we are social animals. We evolved to be members of a tribe; when we feel left out, it signals to our bodies that we are in danger. Fight or flight takes over. Inflammation rises.

"Loneliness is a public health problem in western nations," Ravella told me. "Loneliness is one of the biggest stressors that we face in the world in terms of things that can inflame your body. It weakens your immunity, and it's a chronic stressor."

Indeed, as the inflammation caused by social isolation ramps up our fight or flight instinct, feeling lonely often causes us to withdraw even more from society. Being isolated makes us fearful of the world and fearful of other people.

And loneliness is also closely linked to Alzheimer's and other forms of cognitive decline. In one study published in 2022, researchers found not only a clear link between social isolation and dementia but also that, among those who had no other risk factors, being lonely *tripled* the risk of developing cognitive decline over the ensuing ten years. It was also associated with poorer executive function, lower brain volume, and greater overall damage to brain tissue.

It's a vicious cycle. Loneliness makes us stressed. Stress causes inflammation. Inflammation makes us withdraw even further. All of it increases our risk of dementia. And at the heart of the struggle?

Your microbiome.

A 2020 study measured a cohort of 655 subjects on a scale of loneliness, wisdom, and compassion. The researchers found that those who had the highest levels of loneliness and the lowest levels of social support also showed the lowest levels of diversity in their microbiome. Other studies have shown that the wider and more diverse your social network, the healthier and more diverse your microbiome, while anxiety and stress are linked to reduced diversity.

"No matter how old we are, or whether we are with a partner or living alone, I think having that social support in whatever form is critical," not just for our mental health, but for the health of our microbiome, said Ravella. "Keep that openness to meeting new people. It's something that should be prescribed in physicians' offices."

HOW TO USE YOUR BRAIN TO CHANGE YOUR GUT—AND VICE VERSA

Although our microbiome can powerfully affect our cognitive function and emotional state, the relationship is mutual, particularly when it comes to how we handle stress.

Consider the relationship between ulcers and stress. Numerous studies in the twentieth century found a link between reported stress levels and the risk of developing an ulcer. Doctors speculated that stress caused an increase in stomach acidity, which caused the stomach to develop holes in its lining.

We've since discovered that, in fact, ulcers are caused by the overgrowth of a specific gut bacterium, H. pylori. When it grows out of control, it can cause a deterioration of the gut lining. But it turns out the original premise that linked stress and ulcers wasn't that far off: More recent research has shown higher levels of stress are linked to overgrowths of H. pylori. So stress does cause ulcers, but not the way we once thought: It causes ulcers by altering our microbiome.

Or consider the relationship between stress and the immune system.

It's accepted wisdom that when you're under stress, you're more likely to catch cold. The reason may center in the gut: Studies of stressed-out college students during finals week found changes to their microbiomes, including a reduction in certain bacteria that help to regulate the immune system.

So, while the health of the microbiome may be one of the biggest factors in the health of your mind, your mind also has a unique ability to heal your microbiome. Control your stress and eat a diverse diet filled with plant fibers, and you control the keys to the microbial kingdom—and improve your odds of staying sharp, focused, and, yes, happy for life.

Seven Ways to Calm Your Microbiome

Stress can figuratively scramble your brain, but it can literally scramble your microbiome. To help you protect yourself, and your 100 trillion best friends, I spoke with Daniel Kirsch, president of the American Institute of Stress, a nonprofit in Weatherford, Texas, to get his best advice on how to chill out fast.

Raise your hand. The best way to stop something from gnawing at you is to open up and let it out. Ask a professional or trusted friend what they think of the problem that's nagging you. You may not solve the problem right away, but that's fine. Simply taking action toward solving it is what will make the difference, Kirsch said.

Take stress breaks. "To charge your phone, you have to plug it in," Kirsch told me. "To charge your brain, you have to unplug it." Take opportunities to focus on just one thing. "When you sit down to eat breakfast, just concentrate on enjoying breakfast. Don't plan the day."

Use the quieting reflex. When something disturbs you, simply relax your jaw and smile, inwardly. Then, take in one deep breath—not an exaggerated breath. (You should be able to do it without anyone in the room noticing.) "Visualize hot air coming up through the bottom of your feet, through your body, and filling your lungs," Kirsch said. This technique should quickly short-circuit an acute stress reaction.

Walk. A long walk in nature would be great, but that's not always available. Fine, Kirsch said. Simply walking around the living room for a little while can help break you out of an ongoing stress cycle.

Get distracted. "Think of a baby crying. To stop them, you give them something new to play with," said Kirsch. When you're in distress, take a moment to look up information on something completely different from what is stressing you out. Make it meaningless: "Who played second guitar on *Frampton Comes Alive*?" (Bob Mayo) "What state has the most greenhouses?" (Pennsylvania).

Make your bed. Admiral William McRaven wrote the book on it, but Kirsch loves the advice. When you start your day by making your bed, you start your day with a feeling of control and accomplishment, he explained.

Be compassionate, not empathetic. Caregivers have double the rate of severe depression as the general population. "It's called compassion fatigue," said Kirsch. "I tell my medical students, 'Don't feel their pain. Leave that to Bill Clinton.' There is a difference between being sympathetic and being empathetic. We need to have sympathy, but we also need to isolate ourselves a bit. We can't allow ourselves to feel others' pain."

6

The Inside Story of Your Belly

The modern world can be an inhospitable place for the ancient microbes that live in your gut. Here's how to protect them, naturally.

If you want to bolster your financial resources, you might go to the bank and apply for a loan. In the years to come, if you want to boost your overall physical health, you may find yourself applying for a loan from a different type of bank.

The poop bank.

I hope they have a competition to come up with a name for the poop bank.

Wells Far-Go Number Two?

JP Morgan Waste?

Something that rhymes with *Citibank*, perhaps?

Actually, there's already an official name for it: The Microbiota Vault, a global effort to collect, analyze, and preserve microbiomes from around the world, is currently being planned as a storage facility built into the side of a mountain in Switzerland.

Storing samples of biological resources to preserve our future health isn't a new idea: The Svalbard Global Seed Vault in Norway collects seed and grain samples from around the world, protecting them from extinction. The Microbiota Vault will do the same.

Except it's not food they're collecting. It's poop.

The idea of a bank to store feces seems odd at first, but less so when you consider the enormous role that the microbes in our guts play in our overall health—and what seems to be happening to those microbes.

A few years ago, scientists gathered up fossilized fecal matter from caves in the American Southwest. The dry atmosphere and the darkness of the caves had contributed to preserving these remnants of the hunter-gatherers who lived in their recesses up to two thousand years ago—or at least, the remnants of their bowel movements—allowing researchers to extract DNA from the fossilized fecal matter. In addition, the researchers also collected contemporary fecal samples from people around the globe, from industrialized city dwellers to nomadic tribes in Africa. They then compared the caveman poop to the samples collected from around the modern world.

The researchers found that most species of bacteria that appeared in the millennia-old samples were also found in the samples taken from today's nomadic tribes. But a whopping 39 percent of the species found in the cave remains were completely missing from the microbiomes of people living in today's industrialized societies. "[T]he industrial human microbiome has diverged from its ancestral state," the researchers concluded.

It's not a new finding. Researchers have been sounding the alarm about the lack of diversity in our microbiomes for the past few decades.

"In 2009 we published a paper that found that the problem with the microbiome is that we are losing diversity by generation," Maria Gloria Dominguez-Bello, PhD, microbiologist at Rutgers University, told me recently. "And in the fifteen years since we published, the issue has only gotten worse."

Hence the need for a poop bank. You may see what you leave behind as inert waste, but more than half of your poop is actually alive—it's made up of living microbes. (The majority of the rest of it is discarded cells from your digestive tract.) Researchers speculate that one day we may discover that a specific set of microbes is essential to treat or prevent certain diseases and that, as our natural microbiome is destroyed, we will need to go back in time to recover those microbes of centuries past and find ways to reintroduce them into the human body.

In fact, scientists argue, that lack of microbial diversity is already wreaking havoc on our health, our fitness—and our weight.

THE NATIONAL FOREST IN YOUR BODY

Imagine your body as a great national park, a Yosemite of You.

The trillions of bacteria, viruses, and fungi living on and inside of your body represent somewhere in the vicinity of ten thousand unique species, all of which play specific roles in managing your health. Many of these species thrive in abundance, growing gleefully in your gut; others are lurkers, remaining in small numbers until an opportunity arises for them to bloom. These microbes cling to the walls of your digestive tract and, in doing so, make it difficult for pathogens and less-healthy microbes to find a place to set up shop. They break down indigestible food fibers, creating short-chain fatty acids (SCFAs) that help to regulate our immune systems; balance our hormones (including those that control insulin sensitivity, hunger, and satiation); and create energy used by the cells in the liver and muscles. They manufacture vitamins, help control blood pressure, even metabolize drugs.

These ten thousand unique, diverse species live in harmony, interacting with one another—and with you, their host—in ways that science is only beginning to understand. When that diversity is disturbed—because of a change in diet, the introduction of unhealthy pathogens, or a chemical that damages the microbiome—the results can be wildly unpredictable.

In his book *Missing Microbes*, infectious disease specialist Martin Blaser, MD, explains how changing even one aspect of a diverse eco-system can have dramatic, unexpected, long-term consequences:

> [W]hen wolves were removed from Yellowstone National Park seventy years ago, the elk population exploded. Suddenly it was safe for elk to browse on, and ultimately denude, the tasty willows that line most riverbanks. Songbirds and beavers that depended on willows to nest and build dams dwindled in number. As the rivers eroded, waterfowl left the region. With no wolf-kill

carcasses to scavenge, ravens, eagles, magpies and bears declined. More elk led to fewer bison due to competition for food. Coyotes came back to the park and ate the mice that many birds and badgers relied on. And so on, down a dense web of interactions perturbed when a keystone species was removed. This concept holds true in the natural world as well as your microbiome . . .

Forage for Your Porridge

On spring, summer, and especially fall evenings, when I take our dog, Travis, for a walk, I'll sometimes bring along a little oiled-cotton pouch, a "foraging bag," my wife gave me. I'll use it to collect some items that grow wild in our neighborhood, which I like to play around with as food. Some, like chives, I could buy in the grocery store, but they spring up wild in our backyard, so I'll cut them up and add them into omelets.

Others are more obscure. Beech nuts (amazing and delicious, like pine nuts) and hickory nuts (impossible to break open, but also delicious, like sweeter versions of walnuts) both grow wild in our area. I can sometimes find purslane, a salty, succulent weed that grows all over the world and is the most potent plant source of omega-3 fatty acids, and I'll add it to salads. And we are blessed with robust wild red raspberry bushes, which yield intense and delicious fruits in mid-July, and with wild blackberries, which aren't quite as delicious but work well as toppings for yogurt or ice cream or fillings for pies.

Most of what Travis and I find on our journeys are plants that are entirely different from the plants that are sold in the grocery store, and as such they help to add to the diversity of our family's microbiomes. There are scores of other plants growing in our neighborhood that could be eaten, if one were particularly adventurous—everything from daylilies to violets to milkweed. For a great, pocket-sized guide to eating your backyard or local woodlands, check out *Peterson Field Guide to Edible Wild Plants.*

It's exactly what is happening inside each and every one of us. But instead of denuded willows and eroded riverbanks, the damage we're experiencing comes in the form of skyrocketing rates of obesity and diabetes. Blaser and Dominguez-Bello outline the connection in their documentary film *The Invisible Extinction,* which you can watch on various streaming services. And the extinction they warn of stems from three enormous changes that have occurred in our environment: the introduction of antibiotics, the widespread use of industrial fertilizers and pesticides, and the reduction in diversity in the diets we consume.

A PRESCRIPTION FOR WEIGHT GAIN

When was the last time you came down with a nasty cold or flu and, after waiting it out for a day or two, gave in, went to the doctor, and got a prescription for antibiotics?

A few days after starting those antibiotics, you probably experienced some relief from your symptoms. The antibiotics worked! Science is amazing!

Well, science is amazing, but so is the human body. And in the vast majority of cases, it was the natural healing power of your immune system, not the antibiotics you got from your doctor, that knocked out your cold. In fact, at least one in three prescriptions for antibiotics given to humans is entirely useless, according to the Centers for Disease Control and Prevention; they're broad-spectrum (read: kill everything) antibiotics prescribed for colds and flus—illnesses that are caused by viruses and against which antibiotics have no power.

Prescriptions can provide powerful antidotes to our health issues, but they also have a tremendous placebo effect; when we take them, we attribute any subsequent change in our wellbeing to the drugs we took, rather than to the natural healing process of the body. We want the doctor to give us something that will make us feel better, fast.

But while those antibiotics don't help us get over our colds any faster, they have a profound effect on our bodies; when they get into our system, they create mass extinction events within our

microbiomes. And much like the eroding rivers caused by the elim-
ination of wolves in Yellowstone, there's no telling what the long-
term, downstream effects of antibiotics will be on your microbiome
and on your health.

For example, "When was the last time a doctor told anyone, 'If you
take antibiotics, it could increase your risk of diabetes'?" Blaser asked
me during a recent interview. Well, that is exactly what happens: In
a Danish study of more than one million people, investigators found
that people who had type 2 diabetes had used more antibiotics over
the previous fifteen years than those who did not.

Most people don't think about antibiotics as drugs that make you
gain weight and become diabetic, but the science isn't exactly new:
The relationship between antibiotics and weight gain was established
seventy-five years ago, when farmers observed that by feeding their
pigs, chickens, and cows antibiotics, the animals would grow fatter,
faster. The same technique is used in just about every kind of animal
husbandry today; from the turkey on your Thanksgiving plate to the
lox on your bagel, most every commercial animal protein has been
forced to grow fat with antibiotics.

So, if antibiotics make animals fat, why wouldn't they have the
same effect on us?

They do. A 2021 review of literature on antibiotics and weight gain
in the journal *Metabolism* found that "[D]espite their undoubted use-
fulness, there is now a growing body of evidence that these agents may
contribute to the development of obesity via alterations in the gut
microbiota."

Another review of studies that same year, published in *Current
Obesity Reports,* found that the administration of antibiotics early in
life, repeated exposure to antibiotics for three or more courses, and
treatment with broad-spectrum antibiotics were all associated with
increased odds of obesity. And a New Zealand study looked at more
than 151,000 children and found that when their mothers took antibiotics during pregnancy, or when the children were given antibiotics
in the first two years of life, there was a greater chance that those children would be obese by age four.

Why does this happen? Well, imagine what happens when a forest is destroyed by a wildfire. Everything is wiped out—trees and bushes, birds and mammals, insects and reptiles, fungi and bacteria. The verdant expanse is turned into a dried-out husk. But it doesn't stay that way.

Scorched soil can't support the vast array of trees that once grew in the forest, so hardscrabble bushes and grasses, their seeds carried in on the wind, start to take over. Critters that can live on and in these scrubby new growths may return, but the owls, eagles, and songbirds that rely on the trees for nests and perches are gone. Instead of a symphony of insects and amphibians singing out at night, only a few creatures that can survive in scrub brush and low-nutrient soil return at first. Without competition from other species, and without natural predators that once lurked in the forest, these species take over, completely altering the terrain. The results are unpredictable, and it may take decades for the forest to return to its healthy, natural state.

That's essentially what happens to the Yosemite of You when you take antibiotics; diversity is wiped out, and the species that either survive the onslaught or recover quickest, the ones that thrive in this new environment, are not necessarily the healthiest. Antibiotics wipe out the songbirds and the sycamores, but the cockroaches and crabgrass linger.

And a dysfunctional microbiome doesn't just cause us to gain weight; it undermines our attempts at losing it. Researchers at the Institute for Systems Biology in Seattle found in 2021 that those with healthy microbiomes responded to weight-loss treatments better than those with unhealthy microbiomes; in fact, they could predict who would successfully lose weight just by looking at the diversity of their gut bacteria.

This book is focused on weight and the effects of the microbiome on obesity. But as we have shown, the microbiome affects every aspect of our health, and the overuse of antibiotics does the same. In 2022 researchers looked at more than 313,000 people and discovered that those who had used antibiotics for ninety-one or more days had a significantly increased risk of Alzheimer's. Other studies have linked the use of antibiotics to everything from colon cancer to kidney stones.

Of course, we shouldn't confuse the damage that antibiotics are capable of with the extraordinary good they can do. Antibiotics are like hammers, automobiles, or vodka: wonderful tools that improve our lives when we use them responsibly. But when mishandled, they can be deadly.

"My specialty is infectious diseases," Blaser told me. "In early COVID I was planting potatoes in our backyard. One day, I realized I had a big bull's-eye lesion on my flank, and it was clear that I had Lyme disease. I did not hesitate to take antibiotics. They are wonderful when used for particular illnesses."

But we have fallen in love with the idea of antibiotics being the cure for all our woes. Internet and over-the-counter sales have made them easier to access. But we need to be more skeptical, even when our docs want to prescribe them.

"Ask your doctor, 'Is this really necessary? Could the infection be viral?'" recommended Dominguez-Bello. "Make the doctor think twice."

Still, you could give every doctor the stiff-arm when it comes to antibiotics, but you can't escape their effect. Because antibiotics, as well as many other man-made substances, are all around us—in our food, our water, our soil, our air. And they may all play a role in our ever-diminishing microbial diversity.

ARE BUG KILLERS KILLING YOUR BUGS?

If your gut is home to trillions of bacteria, fungi, and viruses, then what happens when we expose that microbial biomass to a modern world filled with antibacterials, antifungals, and other chemicals that have been developed to kill off those types of organisms?

Exactly what you'd think would happen.

When researchers studied more than twenty thousand farmers in Thailand, they found that those farmers who worked most frequently with pesticides—including herbicides (weed killers), insecticides, and fungicides—were more likely to be obese and to have diabetes, high cholesterol, and hypertension. Of the thirty-five different pesticides studied, twenty-two were significantly associated with higher obesity.

Many studies have emerged in just the past three years linking insecticides and other pesticides to obesity. And the ways in which those chemicals cause obesity are almost unlimited: They promote fat storage; they prompt stem cells to turn into fat cells; they impact insulin signaling; they alter metabolism; they interfere with hormonal function; they alter our epigenome (the means by which certain genes get turned "on" and "off"); and, yes, they damage the gut microbiota.

It's difficult to control for these environmental factors. More than one billion pounds of pesticides are used in the United States every year, according to the Environmental Protection Agency, with billions more being pumped into our environment annually around the globe. If you are an average American, you have twenty-nine different pesticides inside your body right now, according to the Centers for Disease Control and Prevention. The most common of these is the chemical glyphosate, which you might know as Roundup. In fact, you probably have a plastic jug of it in your garage; it's the most widely used pesticide in the United States. And it has been labeled a threat to your microbiome and, by extension, to your weight, and to your health. "[T]he heavy use of glyphosate-based products may lead to microbial dysbiosis," according to a 2022 Finnish study. "Glyphosate-based herbicides . . . can disrupt the host microbiota and influence human health," researchers wrote in a 2021 study published in *Scientific Reports*.

Glyphosate—which countries from Italy to Vietnam to Qatar have already banned—is used by commercial farmers to grow just about every commercial crop in the United States. In fact, it is found in about 90 percent of American-grown food products—the FDA has even found it in honey. Still, even if it is found in much of our food, limiting your personal exposure makes sense; you may want to think twice before spraying your dandelions with it this summer.

Fortunately, awareness of the impact of pesticides on the obesity epidemic in America is growing: In 2022 the United States joined the European Union in banning the pesticide chlorpyrifos; studies have shown that the chemical disrupts the microbiome, damages the lining of the gut, and "promotes obesity and insulin resistance."

Eating organic whenever possible can help reduce our overall pesticide exposure, but it's not a viable alternative for all of us all of the time: Organic produce can be expensive and often hard to find. But there are other ways to reduce the amount of harmful pesticides you and your family consume. For example, *Consumer Reports* has a tool that allows you to select the produce you're buying and shows which country of origin delivers the lowest pesticide load for that type of fruit or vegetable. What's great about this tool is that it accounts not just for the amount of pesticides used, but for the safety of the particular pesticides. You can learn, for example, that cantaloupe grown in Honduras or Mexico rate "VERY LOW" in pesticide risk, while the same fruit grown in the United States rates a "HIGH" risk. (To find the tool, you can search "consumer reports pesticides in produce," or type in this link: consumerreports.org/cro/health/natural-health /pesticides/index.htm)

As a general rule, I try to buy organic when I'm purchasing foods that I eat without peeling: green vegetables, berries, apples, peppers. I don't bother with organic bananas or avocados, since the skin of the plant helps to create a protective barrier.

But when push comes to shove, I eat whatever plants I can get my teeth into. As David Katz, MD, former director of Yale University's Yale-Griffin Prevention Research Center and founder of Diet ID, recently told me, "Eating organic is healthier. But it is more important to eat a variety of plants than it is to eat organic."

DIY Pesticide-Proofing

Even organic produce will probably carry some trace level of pesticides, so it makes sense to wash all fruits and vegetables before eating. To make cleaning both fast and convenient, combine 1 tablespoon lemon juice, 2 tablespoons distilled white vinegar, and 1 cup cold tap water in a spray bottle. Shake well and spray, then rinse well with tap water. Lemon juice is a natural disinfectant, while white vinegar can neutralize most pesticides.

"The single most important thing is to eat enough fiber," Dominguez-Bello told me. "Fibers from fruits and vegetables are the food for our microbes. Diversity drives diversity. If you only eat one type of fiber, you're only going to feed one type of microbe." Indeed, Dominguez-Bello and Blaser, who are a couple in their personal lives as well as research partners, put a great deal of effort into maximizing their dietary diversity.

"Gloria is the main cook in our house, but there are three foods that I make," Blaser said. "Every day I make a fruit smoothie that has seven or eight different fruits. That's meal number one. Then I make yogurt with some kind of grain plus seven or eight different fruits, mostly berries. Then a salad which has five or six different vegetables. So each day we are eating twenty different plants."

Makes getting just thirty in seven days sound pretty slacker, no?

7

Put Those Damn Vitamin Pills Down—Now!

Your 100 trillion microbes know what they want from your food. But they can't make heads or tails out of those pills in your pantry.

have amazing news. I've just created a pill. A very special pill. I'm selling it online, in vitamin stores, at your local pharmacy, and even in the health section of your supermarket. And I think this pill will be very good for you. You should take it every day—for the rest of your life.

Before giving you the pill, however, I'll provide you with a few important caveats: First, the pill is expensive—figure about $40 a month, minimum—and not covered by insurance. Second, you'll be receiving no medical testing or guidance, nor will there be any way to monitor the pill's effect on your body, positive or negative. Third, there is no solid scientific evidence that said pill will have any positive effect on your health whatsoever, and some experts have expressed concern that it might actually be harmful. And fourth, because there is no government oversight, there's no way to guarantee that what I say is in the pill is, in fact, actually in the pill.

Ready to invest lots of dough in this exciting new supplement?

Mmmm . . . maybe you'll take a pass on that one.

But if you regularly consume a multivitamin or an individual supplement not recommended by your doctor, then you've already said yes to the rather specious offering above. And you're not alone: One study found that 70 percent of American adults take at least one vitamin or supplement daily, and almost three in ten take four or more. Multivitamins, vitamin D, and omega-3 fatty acids are the most common nutritional pills we pop, and, according to the research firm Zippia, the average American who uses supplements is now dropping about $500 a year on them.

The supplement business is a great business—as long as you're on the sales side, that is. Because supplements are not regulated by the government, there are no annoying scientific studies to fund, no quality control issues to worry about, no ongoing research to stay on top of. Just put something into a pill, label it a "nutritional supplement," and put it on the drugstore shelf: It's so simple that there are more than 29,000 nutritional supplements on the market today, with 1,000 more being added every year. And why not: The average profit margin on a line of supplements is a whopping 38 percent. *Cha*-freakin'-*ching*.

Yet the United States Preventive Services Task Force (USPSTF), the scientific body authorized by Congress to review scientific evidence around preventive medical services, says that "the current evidence is insufficient to assess the balance of benefits and harms of the use of multivitamin supplements, or single or paired nutrient supplements." So while Americans will shell out an estimated $56.7 billion for these pills and powders in 2024, there's little if any evidence that we're actually doing ourselves any good.

Increasingly, it's starting to look like we might be causing our bodies harm.

How is this possible? Let's take a closer look.

VITAMIN PILLS: LIKE LEECHES, BUT WITHOUT ALL THE BLOOD

Imagine you're stuck at home, bored to tears, with no way of getting around town. Now let's say you read about a scientific study that found 100 percent of people who successfully drive themselves around town do so while holding a steering wheel. This would seem to be irrefutable evidence! And there's an ad for steering wheels right there in your Facebook feed!

So you click on the ad, order a steering wheel, and in a few days a box arrives at your house. You unwrap your new steering wheel, grab hold with both hands, and go . . . nowhere.

Was the study wrong? No, but while the evidence is irrefutable that people who successfully drive around town use a steering wheel, there's a heck of a lot of information left out of that sentence. Like, for example, the fact that the steering wheel needs to be attached to a car.

This sounds ridiculous, but it's not unlike how we treat research around vitamins and minerals. We have a lot of information about little, tiny bits of the puzzle, but our overall understanding of the larger issue is still pretty fuzzy. But a little piece of the puzzle is all anyone needs to market a product.

Vitamin E, for example, is an important nutrient that science has repeatedly linked to improved long-term cognition and heart health. And vitamin E is hard to get from food, since it's mostly found in nuts and seeds—plentiful in the supermarket, but a food group that many of us neglect. It would seem to make sense that if you want a healthy heart and a healthy brain, you should invest in a daily vitamin E pill.

Except . . .

Vitamin E, in its natural state, is composed of an array of different chemicals called tocopherols. Which of these chemicals is the most bioactive? Which ones protect us from harm? How do these different substances work together? How much of each do we need? Science doesn't actually know, but that won't stop vitamin manufacturers from charging you somewhere between $20 and $40 for a bottle of vitamin E pills. What we do know is that the most common form of vitamin E supplement, called a-tocopherol, has been shown to reduce blood levels of y-tocopherol, another form of the vitamin. One study has found that while a-tocopherol can reduce the risk of Alzheimer's, it only does so in the presence of y-tocopherol.

So, are those E pills hurting, helping, or doing nothing? There's simply no way to tell. One review of research on vitamin E looked at twenty-two different studies. Of those twenty-two studies, eleven found vitamin E was protective, and eleven found that it wasn't. The researchers concluded that we should probably be getting vitamin E from plants and that toxicity levels have not been fully established, so taking the vitamin in supplement form may present certain health risks. Because vitamin E can also act as a blood thinner, combining it with other drugs or with intense bouts of exercise can even prove fatal, Nir Barzilai, MD, founding director of the Institute for Aging Research at Albert Einstein College of Medicine in New York, recently pointed out.

As a general rule, "Vitamin E in pill form does not work," said Katherine Tucker, PhD, director of the Center for Population Health at the Zuckerberg College of Health Sciences at University of Massachusetts, Lowell. We don't fully understand why: It might be that we need a balance of these tocopherol compounds. Or it might be that vitamin E doesn't work unless it's consumed in combination with the polyphenols, fibers, and polyunsaturated fatty acids that are found in nuts. Or there might be another, as-yet-unknown reason. But when you buy a bottle of vitamin E supplements, you're essentially buying the steering wheel. You're not buying the car. Worse, you might be undermining the benefits of the healthy foods you actually are eating.

It boils down to this: As it digests plant fibers, the microbiome produces essential nutrients—including vitamins and polyphenols—in ways that the human body, without those 100 trillion assistants, simply can't do. It's entirely possible, then, that the process of extracting nutrients from food by way of the microbiome plays a significant role in our bodies' ability to use those nutrients, and hence a pill that offers a synthetic version of a specific nutrient, but gives the microbiome nothing to do, is simply a waste. Our bodies—informed and driven by our microbiome—instinctively know what nutrients to take from food, and how to use those nutrients to protect our health.

Our bodies do not know what to do with pills.

And pills simply can't offer us the range of nutrients our bodies need—because science hasn't even identified them all yet. "You want not only the vitamins and minerals" that are found in fruits, vegetables, and whole grains, Tucker told me, "but also the phytochemicals and fiber as well." More than one thousand different phytochemicals have been identified so far, and we have no idea how many more might exist. But we do know that a vitamin E pill doesn't contain one thousand or one hundred or ten or even one of these essential and mysterious additional nutrients that are critical for our health.

But wait . . . isn't vitamin E an important antioxidant? Don't antioxidants prevent aging? You know, scouring for "free radicals" and all that?

Antioxidants like vitamins E, C, and A were all the rage in the 1980s and into the 1990s, but you don't hear much about them today. Why is that? Well, it turns out that the science behind free radicals was pretty shaky to begin with.

What we used to term "free radicals" are more commonly known today as reactive oxygen species (ROS), which researchers have concluded do more than just cause oxidative stress on the body. A review of more than five hundred scientific papers published in *Dose-Response* found that these substances are crucial to a number of processes in the body that help to maintain vibrancy and improve mitochondrial function. Yes, antioxidants are part of our natural food chain, and they perform important tasks within our body, as long as we're eating them in conjunction with the rest of the whole plants they come packaged in. But, the researchers concluded, when it comes to supplements, "antioxidants are useless or even harmful."

INTO THE MULTIVITAMINVERSE

Indeed, no pill manufacturer knows what foods you eat, what medications you take, what your family or personal health background may be. So, no marketer can tell you what supplements you should take, or how those supplements will affect your body.

Still, it's never a bad idea to have a little extra insurance. So, what about a multivitamin? Can't hurt, could help, right?

"Multivitamins are really good . . . for the economy," joked Barzilai, author of *Age Later: Health Span, Life Span, and the New Science of Longevity*. "I used to think, *Who cares?* Because some of those vitamins don't have what they say they have anyhow. But for some people, they can be dangerous. Many supplements can be linked to increased aging."

Indeed, evidence on multivitamins has been conflictual for decades. A 2023 study linking multivitamins to a reduced risk of Alzheimer's disease got plenty of play in the media. But even the lead researcher of that study, neurologist Adam Brickman, PhD, of Columbia University, warned against relying on supplements: "Supplementation of any kind shouldn't take the place of more holistic ways of getting the same micronutrients," he said in the accompanying press release. "Though multivitamins are generally safe, people should always consult a physician before taking them."

A similar study of 5,947 men sixty-five and older found that after twelve years of consistent multivitamin use, there was no evidence of any benefit to their long-term cognitive function, nor was there any reduction in the risk of age-related cognitive decline. In an editorial in the journal *Annals of Internal Medicine* titled "Enough Is Enough: Stop Wasting Money on Vitamin and Mineral Supplements," Johns Hopkins researchers cited a large review of studies covering 450,000 people that found no benefit to supplements in terms of reducing risk of heart disease or cancer.

"There's no such thing as one pill fits all," agreed David Sinclair, PhD, anti-aging researcher, professor of genetics at Harvard University, and author of *Lifespan: Why We Age—and Why We Don't Have To.* "A lot of the supplements that are out there, especially multivitamins, have some components that are not only unnecessary but can be dangerous if taken every day," he told me. "An example of that is iron; of course, some women at certain times of the month need more iron, but in general higher levels of iron do associate with increased cellular senescence, which is a hallmark of aging. So I'm wary of people taking multivitamins every day."

"I don't generally suggest people take a multivitamin," agreed Florida Atlantic University's Richard Isaacson, who previously founded the Alzheimer's Prevention Clinic at Weill Cornell Medicine Center in New York. "We should always try to get the vitamin or mineral from diet first." With his patients, Isaacson does extensive, long-term testing of their blood levels of various nutrients, and that information, combined with a lengthy health history and nutritional overview, may determine whether or not he recommends any particular supplement.

For example, if a patient's bloodwork shows low levels of omega-3 fatty acids, "I'll recommend they eat fish. And if they're eating fish several times a week, and their omega-3 levels barely go up, then yes, they may need a supplement. But that, I hope, is where the field is headed: 'Which exact vitamins and supplements and drugs might help you as an individual?'

"My recommendation is, talk to your primary care doctor. If you're really interested in nutritional supplements, ask for a recommendation to a preventative care specialist—a doctor who will have the time to do the testing and to spend time with you to understand your specific needs."

THE TOXIC DETOX

Yikes! If, like most Americans, you've been popping vitamin pills like Skittles, you might be a little concerned by this emerging medical consensus about supplements. You might even think you need to "detox" your body—especially your liver—from all those antioxidants you've been scarfing down.

But please, don't. Few things available over the counter are as toxic as "detoxes."

In fact, a 2016 analysis from the National Institutes of Health and the American Association for the Study of Liver Disease found that approximately one in five cases of liver toxicity in the United States is caused by herbal supplements, many of which were taken in an attempt to lose weight, build muscle, or "cleanse" the liver. The majority of those injuries are from "multi-ingredient nutritional supplements"—that is, pills and potions marketed as cure-alls that are mashups of various herbs linked to weight management or liver health (often through folklore, rather than through science). The researchers explained that it was impossible to know which of the herbal ingredients were the cause of the damage—or whether the injury was caused by a combination of herbs or by some other contaminant that was found in the product. However, they did call out one ingredient—

green tea extract—as both a common ingredient in liver detoxes and a leading cause of liver damage.

Despite all the reports of this substance causing liver damage, there are still dozens of varieties of green tea extract on the market, all with fuzzy and sometimes contradictory medicinal promises. GNC claims its green tea extract (approximately 4 cents a pill) "supports metabolism." (Which is true, but so does nearly every other food or drink on the face of the earth.) Thorne claims its green tea product, at 50 cents a pop, has a "thermogenic (fat-burning) effect." (True again, but everything else you ingest will have a thermogenic effect.)

But wait, there's more . . . Pure Encapsulations markets green tea extract that supposedly "supports neurocognitive, cardiovascular, and cellular health"—a bargain at just 2.4 cents per pill. Life Extension says its green tea pill (about 4.4 cents a dose) does all that plus "helps maintain cholesterol levels." And Renue says its green tea capsules "suppress the activity of pro-inflammatory chemicals produced in your body," for just under 50 cents a pill.

If the people selling us this stuff can't even agree on what it does . . . what the heck are we doing shelling out money for this? And more important, what the heck is it all doing to our bodies? University of Rochester Medical Center experts warn that green tea extract can reduce the effectiveness of blood pressure and heart medications, including beta-blockers and blood thinners. Side effects of green tea supplements can include jaundice (yellowing of your skin or eyes), nausea, and stomach pain.

I've picked on green tea extract here, but there are many, many supplements that can have negative side effects, and very, very little evidence that supplements can have a positive impact on your health.

But you know what can definitely have a positive impact on your health, your weight, and your mood?

Eating more plants.

Are There Any Supplements I *Should* Take?

In general, we need to think plants, not pills. Nutrients that come from within the structure of food are generally more accessible, less expensive, and come with a side serving of other important nutrients. But there are three supplements that the health-conscious person should seriously consider taking—after a talk with his or her doctor.

Vitamin D: As little as ten to fifteen minutes in a sunny window gives you all the vitamin D you need. But as we age, our ability to turn sunlight into vitamin D begins to fade. So, too, does the amount of time we spend outdoors. And vitamin D—which is actually a hormone—is hard to get from food. It's typically found in fatty fish like sardines; we used to get D from our animals, but today most farm animals are raised indoors, away from the nurturing sunlight. Some dairy products and juices are supplemented with D, but if you don't drink milk, there is a chance that you might be among the estimated one in four Americans who have low levels of vitamin D.

Vitamin D is critical for maintaining brain health and bone health, since D helps to direct the use of calcium in the body. So, a D3 supplement might make sense for you. But, Isaacson told me, you should have a blood test to measure your levels of D, and take supplements only under the direction of a doctor.

Calcium: Throughout this book, I recommend dairy repeatedly, and for good reason: It's not just the best but often the only source of calcium for the average American. (About 72 percent of the calcium Americans consume comes from dairy.) Some plants, especially cruciferous vegetables like kale, collard greens, and broccoli, have small amounts. And if you eat a lot of small, boney fish like anchovies, you're getting extra calcium from the little bones you're ingesting. But unless your diet is very different from the average person's, hanging your health on whether you eat enough collard greens and anchovies is probably not an effective long-term strategy.

Adults should get at least 1,000 milligrams (mg) per day; women over fifty and men over seventy should graduate to about 1,200 mg daily. And that's quite a bit: A cup of milk has about 300 mg; a scoop of whey protein powder has about 160 mg. A slice of cheddar gives you another 200. So getting to 1,000 to 1,200 mg per day means you'll need to be eating and drinking a lot of dairy, or you might want to talk with your doctor about a supplement.

Vitamin B12: This B vitamin is essential for maintaining brain health and nerve function. But unless you're vegan, you probably get plenty of B12 already. Animal products like meat, fish, poultry, cheese, and eggs are all rich in the nutrient.

So why is it on this list? As we age, our bodies may have difficulty absorbing vitamin B12 because we begin to produce less stomach acid. Antacids and diabetes medications can also interfere with our B12 absorption. If you're over sixty-five, it's worth discussing with your doctor and asking for a blood test to check your levels. But please, do not just go willy-nilly and start swallowing B12. Federal dietary guidelines call for a daily intake of 2.4 micrograms for all adults, yet some pills come with as much as 1,000 micrograms per dose. It's not clear how taking nearly 500 times as much of this vitamin as you need might hurt you.

8

Eat This Program . . . Anywhere!

***Whether it's a romantic anniversary dinner
at the local French food palace or a quick
trip to the down-and-dirty drive-thru, this
handy cheat sheet makes it easy to pick the
perfect meal every time.***

When it comes to eating the best possible diet for your microbiome, there are two immutable rules:

1. You're almost always better off cooking at home, and
2. You can't always cook at home

As we've learned in previous chapters, among the primary enemies of your microbiome—and hence your body's ability to manage inflammation, prevent weight gain, and improve overall health—are ultra-processed foods. The fewer processed foods in your diet, the better.

Yet while it's relatively easy to avoid processed foods at home—what you don't buy, you can't eat—even restaurants that serve relatively healthy offerings often use highly processed fats like soybean or vegetable oils, and a surprising number of foods on the menu of even mom-and-pop restaurants come premade, prepackaged, frozen, and ready for the deep fryer. Those chicken wings, jalapeño poppers, fried wontons, onion rings, and sweet potato fries? In many cases, they're shipped in from a wholesaler, tossed into a vat of boiling soybean oil, and served—at a serious markup—as "hand-cut" or "homemade." Most salad dressings, waffle batters, and smoothies also come from factory-made mixes. These products are the very definition of "processed."

All of this makes your belly bugs very unhappy. And if your goal is to protect your microbiome, helping it do its job of lowering inflammation and sparking weight loss, then navigating the world of restaurants means doing a little bit of preplanning.

That's where this chapter comes in.

If you know a few simple tricks, it's relatively easy to get around the challenges of most restaurants—whether it's a fast-food franchise, a mid-level sit-down chain, a local diner, or your neighborhood ethnic specialty joint. Pull up a seat, grab a fork, and let's chow down on some useful information.

THE MEXICAN CANTINA

Latin-American cuisine is among the healthiest food on the planet—assuming you're eating it in Latin America, where plant-rich platters, fresh fish, and legumes dominate. But once that food starts gravitating north of the border, a strange thing happens: Everything either gets dumped into a deep fryer or wrapped in a tortilla the size of a parachute.

The worst offenders are the Mexican fast-food and fast-casual chains. For example, fish tacos would sound like a smart choice for someone looking to eat healthfully. But On the Border's Dos XX Fish Tacos will deliver you 1,950 calories (a full day's worth) and 3,549 milligrams of sodium—more than double what the American Heart Association would like you to eat in a day. On the Border of what? A stroke?

If you're craving Mexican, you're almost always better off skipping the big chains and visiting your local cantina, where far more healthful meals are on tap. To land a perfect meal:

- Get that guacamole. Avocados are high in fiber and heart-healthy, brain-healthy monounsaturated fats. Many restaurants offer variations like pomegranate, hot peppers, or pineapple that allow you to add even more plants into this artery-clearing appetizer.
- Swap flour for corn tortillas. Authentic Mexican tacos are made from soft corn tortillas, which are nothing but whole grain corn and water. Flour tortillas, the bastardized American version, are made from white flour and lard, contain up to 300 (empty!) calories, deliver zero fiber, and have more carbs than three slices of bread.
- Keep mole holy. This rich, dark sauce is made from chocolate, chilies, nuts, and spices. That's a lot of Power Plants!
- Check out the rice and beans. If they're serving brown rice and whole beans, you couldn't order a healthier side dish. If they're serving white rice and refried (that is, cooked in lard) beans, take a pass.
- Think vegetarian nachos. Many places offer nachos topped with grilled vegetables, beans, guac, sliced jalapeños, and other whole plants. You can add meat and cheese as you see fit, but if you're getting meat with your main meal, you don't need it in the nachos.

What to avoid: Anything that comes in a fried tortilla, including the taco salad, which is usually iceberg lettuce, ground beef, and cold, sad tomatoes in a big bowl of deep-fried, empty calories. Also avoid burritos of any kind, unless you're planning to eat what's inside and leave the big white-flour tortilla on your plate.

THE GREAT AMERICAN DINER

There's nothing better on a Sunday morning than sliding into a diner booth, whether it's to satisfy the appetite you worked up in church, or because you still haven't made it home from Saturday night's festivities. Regardless of the state of your soul and/or liver, the gloriously greasy diner is one of America's great contributions to the world's cuisine.

The prime drawback with diners, however, is that there aren't many plants on the menu. But you can find them if you look.

- Start with an omelet. This is generally the best place to sneak in veggies, even if it's little more than peppers and onions or spinach. But with the eggs and cheese, you're getting protein as well as fiber from the vegetables. Add a fruit cup and you're starting your day in pretty good shape.
- Or the oatmeal. Top it with fresh berries if they have 'em, raisins if they don't. Avoid brown sugar, maple syrup, and "craisins," which are cranberries coated in sugary syrup.
- Seek out whole wheat. Sometimes "wheat" bread is just white bread that's been dyed with molasses to make it darker. Ask if the diner offers 100 percent whole wheat bread or even a whole wheat bagel or English muffin.
- Get buckwheat, dammit! Some diners will offer buckwheat pancakes, which are a whole different game from your standard pancake. Buckwheat is gluten free, high in fiber, and a complete protein—the breakfast version of quinoa. Boom! Power Plant number one.

What to avoid: In the hierarchy of carbohydrate evil, waffles are the top offender, often weighing in north of 500 calories; white-flour pancakes deliver about 165 empty calories; French toast, about 150. If you can get your French toast with 100 percent whole grain bread, that's your ticket. And before you order the muffins, take a look in the display case and see how much grease has oozed out onto the paper. Now imagine it oozing out into your arteries.

THE PIZZA PARLOR

In Italy, pizza is usually an appetizer. In America, it's a main meal.

Unfortunately, it's almost impossible to get enough vegetables and protein onto a couple of slices of pizza to really qualify as a healthy lunch or dinner. That's why you should consider a pie as a part of your overall meal, not the whole thing.

- Keep your crust thin. The thinner the crust, the fewer empty calories you're ingesting. Avoid the Sicilian or Chicago-style versions. At the Chicago-style Uno Pizzeria & Grill, the lowest-calorie "individual" pizza—the healthy-sounding "Farmer's Market"—weighs in at 270 calories per slice, or 1,620 calories per serving, with 90 grams of fat and more than 2,000 milligrams of sodium.
- Praise Caesar. A Caesar salad with grilled chicken is the perfect solution to the pizzeria problem. Tons of fiber, tons of protein, and a perfect accompaniment to a slice or two of pizza pie.
- Know your sauces. Tomato or pesto sauces are almost always the healthiest choice on the menu at any Italian restaurant. Alfredo is almost always the worst.

What to avoid: Almost everything else. Even something that sounds healthy, like eggplant parm, is going to be breaded and fried in oil. Appetizers? Most are breaded and fried in oil. Chicken cutlets? Breaded and fried in oil. Garlic knots? They're just giant fistfuls of empty carbs coated in butter. And be careful of meats: Most Italian offerings are highly processed, like pepperoni, sausage, salami, or capicola. So even an antipasto salad is giving you something your microbiome isn't going to like.

THE CHINESE RESTAURANT

General Tso was a noted Chinese warrior and statesman from the 1600s. But chances are he'd be horrified at the bread- and sugar-encrusted American chicken nugget named after him.

Like a lot of what's found on Chinese restaurant menus in the United States, General Tso's chicken bears little resemblance to anything that's traditionally eaten in China. The same is true of anything labeled "sesame" or "orange," which signifies something sugary, gloppy, and bad for your microbiome. The closer you can get to real Chinese food, the healthier and happier your microbiome will be.

- Divide by two. Why do you have so many leftovers from Chinese food? Because meals in Chinese restaurants are made to serve two. So if you and your partner can't decide on a single entrée, plan on eating just half of what's brought to your table and taking the rest home.
- Embrace the chopsticks. It's a clever way to slow the pace of your eating, allowing time for your brain to get the "I'm full" signal from your belly. You'll be surprised at how many calories (and how much money) you'll save by eating with these tools.
- Seek out the steam. As with almost any cuisine, food that's steamed is going to be healthier than food that's fried. Most of the appetizers on a Chinese menu are deep-fried, but steamed dumplings are a great option for cutting down on the unhealthy grease.
- Swap in the brown rice. Most meat and vegetables are going to be fried, so your best defense is a healthy base on which to spread it all.

What to avoid: Lo mein will lay you low. Even "vegetarian" lo mein means you're primarily eating noodles fried in oil. Fried rice is also a bad idea for the same reason. Anything that's "sweet and sour" is basically a sugar bath.

THE SUSHI SPOT

Often, when ethnically diverse food meets the American palate, terrible things happen. That's not necessarily true with sushi, where some of the most loathed Westernized variations are, in fact, pretty healthy. Consider the much-reviled California roll, with its mix of crab stick,* cucumber, and avocado wrapped in nori, a form of seaweed. That's three plants plus a healthy protein source—bonus plant points if they'll serve it with brown rice instead of white.

---

* What is a "crab stick"? It's typically made of bits of pollock, a sustainable and omega-3–rich cold-water fish, along with some starch and food coloring. So yes, it's processed and hence not as ideal as, say, fresh crab or fresh pollock, but still a solid choice for the occasional meal. (Pollock is also the main ingredient in McDonald's Filet-o-Fish sandwich. Weird, right?)

While freshness is always an issue with sushi (and anyone picking up a plate of raw tuna in a Costco in Kansas ought to know that they're not getting the most authentic of culinary experiences), sushi is usually a microbiome-friendly choice. Here are some ways to amp up your meal:

- Seek out the seaweed salad. It's usually a mix of a few different types of seaweed, topped with sesame seeds. For most of us, that's three or four new, different plants that we typically don't eat. A Power Plant home run, and typically better than the "house salad," which is usually just iceberg lettuce and oily ginger dressing.
- Eat up the edamame. Steamed soybeans are high in both protein and fiber, and they add another Power Plant to your day.
- Focus on the bottom of the food chain. The most popular fish items in the United States are the big predators—salmon, tuna, swordfish. Unfortunately, these fish are also the highest in contaminants, because chemicals accumulate in their bodies as they gobble up schools of smaller sea creatures. By looking around the menu and trying other items like hirame (flounder), hotate-gai (scallop), hokkigai (surf clam), ika (squid), and, my personal favorite, uni (sea urchin), you'll lower your exposure to chemical contaminants. Not a big deal if you eat fish rarely, but if you love sushi, it's important to mix it up.
- Don't sleep on the Spanish mackerel. Also known as saba, this oft-overlooked fish has twice the amount of inflammation-fighting omega-3s as salmon.

What to avoid: Go easy on the soy sauce. A sushi purist knows that a drop or two of soy sauce will do plenty to spice up a piece of fish. If your bowl of soy sauce turns into rice soup halfway through your meal, you're overdoing it—and giving your arteries an unnecessary sodium bath in the process. Also, be aware that "spicy tuna roll" means "tuna roll with a little hot sauce and a lot of mayonnaise." Most commercial mayo is made with soy oil, which is like sticking your tongue in yesterday's deep fryer.

THE THAI RESTAURANT

Thai food feels to many of us like a healthier, lighter version of Chinese food. And while that may be true, if you play your cards poorly, there are many ways you can turn this oft-healthy cuisine into a festival of fat.

- Roll with summer, not spring. Spring rolls are deep-fried, while summer rolls are not.
- Sashay over to satay. Satay is lean grilled meat on a stick, basted with spicy peanut sauce: a great protein base for building your meal.
- Veg out as needed. Most Thai restaurants will offer a combination of tofu and vegetables sautéed in ginger, chiles, and garlic. Order a plate to share, and pack it with as many different plants as you can.
- Get steamed. Most fish at Thai restaurants—and pretty much all restaurants, really—is served deep-fried. But you can often find steamed or broiled fish on the menu, which means you'll get all those great omega-3 fatty acids and far fewer of the processed, unhealthy oils.
- Curry favor with curries. Regardless of color, these dishes are made with coconut milk and vegetables. Pick a lean protein like chicken or shrimp, and see if brown rice is an option.

What to avoid: Anything fried, especially fried rice, which is just empty carbs in oil. Also, rethink noodle-based dishes, which again are primarily empty carbohydrates. (If you crave noodles, get an order of pad Thai and share it, which will get you peanuts and bean sprouts—two more Power Plants!) And stay away from the specialty iced teas and coffees, which are usually loaded with liquid sugar.

THE MIDDLE EASTERN EATERY

Like sushi, this is a cuisine that offers tons of interesting new Power Plants and relatively few pitfalls. To make the most of it,

- Hummus a few bars. Made from ground chickpeas and sesame seeds, plus olive oil (in most quality restaurants—a lot of supermarket brands use cheaper oils), hummus is rich in everything you need, including protein, fiber, and healthy fats. Just go easy with the pitas, which are mostly empty carbs and should be considered nothing more than hummus-delivery devices.
- Bag some baba ghanoush. Chances are you don't eat eggplant very often. Here's a delicious way to get this Power Plant into your weekly diet.
- Put tabouleh on the table. Insanely healthy, this side dish is made of tomatoes, parsley (an underrated nutritional powerhouse), and bulgur, a tasty high-fiber grain.
- Do dessert. Most Middle Eastern desserts are made with honey, butter, and nuts. Good for you? No. Better than most desserts? Definitely. But avoid the Turkish coffee, which is typically served with substantial doses of sugar.

What to avoid: Anything fried in oil, like falafel. While sandwiches like gyros or laffa can be a little high in carbs and calories, they're not terrible choices. But you can do better by getting the meat and vegetables on a platter rather than in a pita. Also, note that shawarma—the meat on a spit roasting at the back of the kitchen—is typically made of fattier cuts, which is why the meat sticks together like that. But geez, it's so good . . .

THE VEGETARIAN RESTAURANT

I recently went on a scuba diving trip in which a big old grouper named Jo-Jo came up to our party and let us pet him under his jaw; later, the fish watched from a distance as we rose back to the surface. I was so moved by the experience that I couldn't eat animals for a few days after that, until the resort served its weekly specialty: grilled grouper.

It was delicious. Sorry, Jo-Jo.

A lot of people are vegetarian-curious, whether for health reasons, concern about the environment, or the simple ethical dilemma of eating creatures that can serve as either meat or pets. But it can be hard to get enough complete protein and enough calcium—two crucial nutrients we need more of as we get older. Plus, not everything that's vegetarian is automatically healthy. See, Skittles. See also, Oreos. Probably not what Gandhi meant when he said man was "born to live on fruits and herbs that the earth grows."

The same holds true in vegetarian restaurants, where you can find plenty of healthy choices, as well as plenty of foods that belong more in the Skittles category.

- Snap up the quinoa and black bean burgers. Most commercial "veggie" burgers are so loaded with preservatives and additives that they're absolutely disqualified from the "healthy" food category. The same goes for Impossible Burgers and other weird meat substitutes. This is not real food; it is processed food, and hence, it's bad for your microbiome. But at many vegan restaurants, the veggie burgers will be made fresh on-site from actual food. Quinoa is a complete protein, which makes it an ideal substitute for animal products.
- Try tempeh. Unlike tofu, tempeh is made from whole soybeans, which means it comes with double the protein of your typical tofu.
- Hail seitan! Made from wheat gluten, seitan does a pretty good job of subbing in for meat, and it works great in stir-fries.

What to avoid: The bread at a "health food" or vegan restaurant is often just as nutrition-free as a baguette or pizza crust; avoid it unless it's explicitly whole grain. The same is true of many desserts; when restaurants take out fat in the form of milk, eggs, and lard, they often replace it with lots and lots of sugar. And don't fall for those fancy "organic" sodas with "natural cane sugar." Sugar is sugar, and it's not good. Look for an unsweetened iced tea or sparkling water.

LE FRENCH BISTRO

While French food has a reputation for being rich in fat, the fact is most bistros offer plenty of lean options. Assuming you don't plan on stuffing a goose's liver down your own throat, there are no shortage of ways to eat healthy.

- Seek out the salads. Although it's usually listed as an appetizer, the Niçoise salad is a perfect meal in itself, loaded with vegetables like green beans, tomatoes, olives, and carrots and topped with an omega-3 rich protein. A number of other salad options, including Salade Parisienne (mixed greens, ham, cheese, potatoes, and egg) and frisée will also up your plant quotient for the week.
- Savor the seafood. Most bistros offer pan-seared fish like salmon, trout, sole, or monkfish.
- Muscle up with mussels. Steak frites can be a celebration of saturated fat, but moules frites (mussels with a side of fries) provides a much leaner meal.

What to avoid: Anything accompanied by the word "confit," which means "to cook slowly in its own fat." And while they're cool and exotic, escargot is just snails in a butter bath, while frog legs are the amphibian form of chicken wings. Worth trying once, but no need to make them a regular part of your meal Français. Crème brûlée is just egg yolks, heavy cream, and sugar. Get it with two spoons or ask for a dessert of berries and cream.

THE INDIAN RESTAURANT

Much Indian cuisine is based around vegetables, and the cooking techniques and array of spices mean you're tasting vegetables in ways you never imagined. Here are some quick options to explore:

- Enter the dal house. A flavorful stew of lentils, dal makes for a great starter or side to your meal.
- Look for vegetarian appetizers. A vegetarian platter will expose you to unique flavors and a wide array of Power Plants.
- Try tandoori. Tandoori entrées are cooked in a tandoor, a traditional clay oven that's the Indian equivalent of a backyard grill—

except that tandoors can reach temperatures of 900°F. Anything tandoori is probably a healthy protein choice.

- Plate some palak paneer. This rich mix of puréed spinach and grilled cubes of cottage cheese is unlike any experience you've had with either of those foods, and a perfect way of getting tons of fiber, protein, and calcium in one mighty dish.

What to avoid: A lot of appetizers on Indian menus are deep-fried. Samosas are small turnovers stuffed with potatoes and then fried. Pakora is battered and deep-fried vegetables.

Amp Up Your Coffee

Coffee shops used to be the purview of private detectives, Beat poets, and the cast of *Friends*. Nowadays, your local Starbucks looks more like a Harry Styles concert, loaded with tweens looking to get an instant watermelon sugar high.

Which has really undercut coffee's position as a healthy beverage. In fact, some scientists estimate that coffee is the number one source of polyphenols in the American diet. And there's a certain type of coffee that's richer in these nutrients than your average cup of joe: espresso. Because it's more concentrated, it packs a more potent polyphenolic punch.

Don't care for the bitter sock in the teeth that espresso packs? Instead of ordering a regular coffee, ask for an Americano. This drink, which is just a shot of espresso mixed with hot water, delivers all the nutritional wallop of espresso in a drink that tastes pretty much identical to regular coffee.

THE "FAST-CASUAL" CHAIN

One of the oddest things about dining out in America is that you can be in Pittsburgh, Plattsburgh, or Phillipsburg and find yourself eating the exact same food from the exact same restaurant with the exact same faux memorabilia on the wall next to your booth. Restaurant chains go to extraordinary lengths to eliminate any geographic or cultural distinctions; Applebee's is the same whether you're visiting Manhattan, New York, or Manhattan, Kansas.

Fortunately, that makes it a lot easier to understand what you're eating. Chain restaurants are required by federal law to post the nutritional content of their meals on their websites. Enter the name of your restaurant and "nutrition menu" into your search bar, and you'll unlock the keys to the kingdom. But it's not going to be pleasant; you'll discover some pretty terrifying truths about your favorite foods—like the fact that, even if you and your date share the Factory Nachos with Spicy Chicken at The Cheesecake Factory, you'll still be downing nearly 1,500 calories *each*. And that's an *appetizer*!

There are, however, plenty of ways to stick a perfect nutritional landing at almost any big sit-down chain. Here's a short list of some smart choices that will give you both the protein your body needs and the Power Plants your microbiome craves:

APPLEBEE'S

Top Sirloin (6 ounces) + Garlicky Green Beans + Steamed Broccoli
440 calories, 5 g fiber, 41 g protein
Blackened Cajun Salmon + House Salad + Signature Cole Slaw
510 calories, 6 g fiber, 42 g protein

CHILI'S

Chicken Enchilada Soup (bowl) + Lunch Combo House Salad + Ranch Dressing (1.5 fluid ounces)
660 calories, 4 g fiber, 24 g protein
Sirloin (6 ounces) + Small Side of Fresh Guacamole + Side of Steamed Broccoli
410 calories, 8 g fiber, 38 g protein

CRACKER BARREL OLD COUNTRY STORE

Lemon Grilled Rainbow Trout + Turnip Greens Bowl
580 calories, 8 g fiber, 67 g protein

OLIVE GARDEN

Grilled Chicken Margherita + Parmesan Garlic Broccoli
540 calories, 6 g fiber, 65 g protein
Herb-Grilled Salmon + Parmesan Garlic Broccoli
460 calories, 5 g fiber, 45 g protein

OUTBACK STEAKHOUSE

Lobster Tail (5 ounces), Steamed (served with fresh mixed veggies
    and seasoned rice) + Sweet Potato
750 calories, 10 g fiber, 32 g protein
Outback Center-Cut Sirloin (6 ounces) + Fresh Steamed Broccoli
360 calories, 5 g fiber, 44 g protein
Steakhouse Salad
750 calories, 7 g fiber, 57 g protein

TEXAS ROADHOUSE

California Chicken Salad
740 calories, 11 g fiber, 78 g protein
Grilled Shrimp House Salad
730 calories, 6 g fiber, 65 g protein
Texas Red Chili (Bowl)
490 calories, 6 g fiber, 35 g protein

FAST-FOOD CHAINS AND DINERS

Dunkin' and Denny's have more in common than just the fact you
can get breakfast at any time of the day. Even though one's primarily a
takeout joint and the other a sit-down diner, they both have the same
goal in mind—getting your food into your stomach as quickly as possible and getting you on your way to make room for the next diner.

The primary drawback of fast food, like diners, is a general lack of
plants on the menu. But with this handy cheat sheet, you can order
quickly and with confidence.

BOSTON MARKET

Turkey Breast (regular) + Bacon Brussels Sprouts + Cornbread
560 calories, 7 g fiber, 39 g protein

BUFFALO WILD WINGS

Brisket Tacos + Slaw
630 calories, 6 g fiber, 32 g protein
Traditional Wings (6) with Signature Sauce + Carrots and Celery
  with Fat-Free Ranch
540 calories, 5 g fiber, 56 g protein

CHICK-FIL-A

Grilled Chicken Sandwich + Kale Crunch Side
560 calories, 7 g fiber, 32 g protein
Spicy Southwest Salad
450 calories, 8 g fiber, 33 g protein

DENNY'S

Loaded Veggie Omelette + Seasonal Fruit + English Muffin
750 calories, 6 g fiber, 34 g protein
Cobb Salad + Wild Alaskan Salmon + Light Italian Dressing
790 calories, 6 g fiber, 53 g protein

DUNKIN'

Kosher Dunkin' Double Veggie Sausage Sandwich
600 calories, 6 g fiber, 37 g protein

IHOP

Egg White Vegetable Omelette w/ Fruit Side
380 calories, 8 g fiber, 29 g protein

JACK IN THE BOX

Chicken Fajita Pita with Salsa + Side Salad + Low-Fat Balsamic
   Vinaigrette
375 calories, 6 g fiber, 28 g protein
Grilled Chicken Salad + Low-Fat Balsamic Vinaigrette
500 calories, 7 g fiber, 26 g protein

KFC

Original Recipe Chicken Breast (on the bone) + Coleslaw
560 calories, 6 g fiber, 40 g protein

McDONALD'S

Premium Asian Salad with Grilled Chicken
270 calories, 5 g fiber, 32 g protein

PANDA EXPRESS

Vegetable Spring Roll (appetizer) + Honey Walnut Shrimp + Super
   Greens
640 calories, 9 g fiber, 22 g protein
String Bean Chicken Breast + ½ order Fried Rice + Super Greens
540 calories, 10 g fiber, 31 g protein

PANERA BREAD

Avocado, Egg White, and Spinach on a Sprouted Grain Bagel Flat
   + Bacon
420 calories, 5 g fiber, 22 g protein
Green Goddess Cobb Salad with Chicken (whole)
530 calories, 8 g fiber, 41 g protein
Turkey on Rustic Sourdough (whole) + Ten Vegetable Soup (cup)
470 calories, 4 g fiber, 32 g protein

POPEYES

Signature Chicken Breast (1) + Cole Slaw (large)
800 calories, 5 g fiber, 38 g protein
Blackened Tenders (5) + Red Beans & Rice (regular)
530 calories, 6 g fiber, 51 g protein

SUBWAY

Turkey and Bacon Guacamole Sub on 9-grain wheat bread with
   lettuce, tomatoes, green peppers, and cucumbers
511 calories, 9 g fiber, 49 g protein
Steak Club Salad
480 calories, 6 g fiber, 45 g protein

TACO BELL

Power Menu Bowl (Chicken)
470 calories, 7 g fiber, 26 g protein
Steak Quesadilla + Black Beans and Rice
690 calories, 8 g fiber, 31 g protein

WENDY'S

Apple Pecan Chicken Salad + Pomegranate Vinaigrette
540 calories, 5 g fiber, 32 g protein
Chili (large) + ½ order Taco Salad
685 calories, 14 g fiber, 37 g protein

9

Muscle Out Fat

*Understanding the secret internal struggle
between fat and muscle, and the smart
strategies that will help the good guys win.*

There's a battle raging inside your body.

There's no fog of war here, no moral ambiguity. There's just an
enemy, bent on death and destruction, and his name is visceral fat. His
primary weapon: inflammation.

But there's a good guy who's fighting to save your life. His name is
muscle. And his secret weapon is the microbiome.

If you can comprehend the stakes of this ongoing conflict, you can
get a pretty good sense of how you should eat and live to stay lean and
healthy: If it's good for your muscles and good for your microbiome,
then do it. If it's not good for your muscles and your microbiome, then
you're just feeding the enemy.

GO AHEAD, MAKE A MUSCLE

Lift your arm, and bend it. Flex that bicep.

The muscle you see when you flex your arm represents about 5
percent of the total skeletal muscle in your body. Now consider this:
That's about how much we lose every decade after age thirty. In other

words, by the time we reach our fifties, the average person loses two armloads of muscle.

This natural process of age-related muscle loss is caused by a combination of various factors, from hormones to a lack of exercise to—yes, you guessed it—inflammation.

Now, if getting healthier and dropping some of the fat from your belly is a top concern for you, then taking care of your muscles might not seem like such a huge priority. Maybe you're not planning on entering an arm-wrestling contest or bodybuilding competition any time soon. Who cares if you're a little lighter in the muscle department?

Well, muscles aren't just for showing off in a T-shirt or helping your neighbor push his car out of a ditch. More muscle—strong, healthy muscle—is vital for many of the things that give you enjoyment in life. When your muscles wither, so do your opportunities to enjoy the world around you. Muscles are essential to keeping you upright and moving, independent and in control, for decades to come.

And it's not exaggerating to say they can save your life.

THE MUSCLE-HEALTH CONNECTION

As we reach middle age, muscle becomes an ever more precious and dwindling resource. Yet think about it: Outside of the occasional strain, sprain, or pain, has your doctor *ever* asked what you were doing to take care of your muscles? Sure, he or she may be concerned about your heart, which is your body's hardest-working muscle. But the *other* muscles in your body are just as important—indeed, the stronger they are, the stronger your heart will likely be. Studies have shown that people with lower muscle mass in their later years have a higher risk of cardiovascular disease. In one study, men with the most muscle mass at age forty-five had an 81 percent lower risk of heart disease than those with the least muscle mass. And if you do have heart disease, staying strong can help you live longer. In a study of people who had been diagnosed with cardiovascular disease, those with higher levels of muscle mass and lower levels of fat had the lowest overall mortality rate.

And it's not just your heart that you're helping:

- Muscle fights hypertension. In a study of men (average age forty-three), researchers found that among those with prehypertension, higher levels of muscular strength were associated with a reduced risk of developing full-blown hypertension in the ensuing years.
- Muscle slashes the risk of metabolic syndrome. Metabolic syndrome refers to a constellation of health issues, including excess abdominal fat, high blood pressure, high blood sugar, and high cholesterol, all of which are tied to heart disease. Several studies have shown that the greater your muscular strength, the lower your chance of developing the syndrome.
- Muscle squelches diabetes. Having more muscle could lower your risk of type 2 diabetes by up to 32 percent, according to one study. Higher muscle mass has also been associated with better insulin sensitivity and lower risk of diabetes or prediabetes; in a study of 13,644 subjects, those with the lowest percentage of muscle were 63 percent more likely to have diabetes than those with the highest percentage.
- Muscle fights off cancer. Breast cancer patients who have high muscle mass have a greater chance of surviving the disease than those who have lower muscle mass, according to a study of 3,241 women (median age fifty-four) with stage 2 or 3 invasive breast cancer. And, in a study of men who had undergone a radical prostatectomy to treat prostate cancer, researchers found that those with the lowest levels of muscle were more likely to see a recurrence of the cancer and more likely to eventually die of the disease.
- Muscle helps prevent Alzheimer's and lowers your risk of dementia. One study looked at 970 older adults who had no evidence of cognitive decline. Researchers put the subjects through a series of strength tests, ranking participants' strength on a scale of −1.6 (weakest) to 3.3 (strongest). Over the next 3.6 years, 15 percent of the subjects developed Alzheimer's. But their risk was strongly determined by where they fell on the strength scale:

For every 1-point increase in muscle strength, a subject's risk of Alzheimer's dropped by 43 percent!

- Muscle makes you smarter. One study found that having low muscle mass was an indicator of low executive function—meaning, the ability to focus, stay organized, and generally run your life. Maybe that "dumb jocks" stereotype doesn't quite hold up!
- Muscle makes you happier. In a study of three thousand adults aged sixty and older, nearly one in ten reported depressive symptoms. The researchers then tested handgrip strength, a common way of measuring overall muscle strength. They found that having a strong grip was inversely related to symptoms of depression; the stronger you are, the less likely you are to become clinically depressed.

For all those reasons and more, it's no wonder low muscle strength is associated with an elevated risk of death, regardless of general health levels, according to a study of 4,449 people aged fifty and older. Even cardio exercise doesn't appear to protect you if you allow your strength levels to deteriorate. The evidence is so clear that a 2019 editorial in the *Journal of Cardiology* recommended that heart doctors start providing their patients with advice on eating and exercising to build muscle.

INFLAMMATION VERSUS MUSCLE: THE ULTIMATE SHOWDOWN

In Chapter 1, we discussed how inflammation plays a major role in weight gain. But it is also a primary driver in the loss of muscle mass as we age. In 2020, a meta-review of hundreds of studies looking at more than 89,000 people found that "higher levels of circulating inflammatory markers are significantly associated with lower skeletal muscle strength and muscle mass."

But the same holds true in reverse: When you build muscle, you lower inflammation and your risk of weight gain. In fact, muscle is a "major immune regulatory organ," according to a 2019 study. No wonder there's a strong connection between healthy muscles and a healthy microbiome: A 2019 review of studies in *Frontiers in Physiology* found that increasing the microbiome's health by feeding it a diverse array of plant fibers can positively impact both muscle mass and physical function.

And our muscles do their best firefighting when we keep them strong. In a creepy but fascinating 2021 study, researchers at Duke University engineered muscle cells in a laboratory, then exposed them to high levels of inflammatory compounds for seven days. As expected, the muscle shrank and became weaker. But when they stimulated the muscle tissue with electrodes to simulate exercise, they discovered the muscle cells directly opposed the pro-inflammatory signaling of the compounds, almost completely wiping out their effects.

So, muscle fights inflammation on its own. But it also fights weight gain in other crucial ways: Muscle sucks up extra blood sugar and stores it in the form of glycogen, which can then be used to power our bodies. The more muscle you have, the more glycogen you can store, and the less of that blood sugar that gets stored in your fat cells. One study found that a low level of muscular fitness was associated with higher odds of gaining at least ten kilograms (twenty-two pounds) over the ensuing twenty years.

Muscle also burns more calories than fat does, even at rest—about six calories a day for a pound of muscle, versus just two calories per day for a pound of fat. That may not seem like a significant difference, but as we get older, that balance means a lot: When we're young adults, muscle can make up about half of our body mass; by age seventy-five, it may be as little as 25 percent.

But fat and chronic inflammation are a devious cabal, and they are not about to take this glucose-storing, immune-system-regulating, calorie-burning interference from your muscles lightly. They have a clever counteroffensive strategy to replace your healthy muscle with flab.

As we saw in Chapter 1, once fat and inflammation take hold, they start to damage the body's insulin receptors. When that happens, more blood sugar gets directed toward the fat cells in the belly, and they continue to swell. Eventually they reach the point of overflow. Fatty acids spill out of the fat cells and flood the rest of the body, accumulating in the liver and the muscles.

This creates a condition called lipotoxicity: As fat builds in the muscles, the muscles themselves begin to lose strength. A study of 1,800 healthy older adults with high levels of intramuscular fat found that while lean muscle mass decreased at about 1 percent per year, strength decreased by up to 4 percent per year.

The stakes in this conflict are high. But maintaining détente between muscles and the microbiome, on one side, and inflammation and belly fat, on the other, is a delicate bit of diplomacy. Because often, when we try to slim down by losing weight, we wind up giving belly fat and inflammation an unexpected leg up.

Fat on the Move!

As babies, we're fat all over. Fat cheeks, fat thighs, fat ankles and wrists. All this subcutaneous fat is there to protect us, providing for what scientists call *homeostasis* but what you and I call keeping it all together. Fat helps to regulate our immune systems, our metabolism, our hormones, our core temperature, and our inflammation levels, ensuring that all of these systems are working together to keep us healthy.

Throughout childhood that fat starts to shift, a change that accelerates at puberty. Our teens and early adulthood are graced by fat falling in all the right places. Even at a woman's leanest, fat makes up 30 to 40 percent of her body; for men that figure is 15 to 20 percent.

And that fat remains protective throughout our lives, even if we start to gain weight in our thighs, our butt, or our love handles—which is why this type of fat, called subcutaneous (or below the skin) fat, isn't linked to such issues as heart disease or diabetes.

So the junk in our trunk is good, but the jelly in our belly is bad. And as we get older, what's in the trunk doesn't want to stay there. Our bodies begin to shift form in middle age; after age forty, visceral fat increases by an average of 200 percent in men, and by 400 percent in women.

Part of this process is simple weight gain. But another significant factor is that, as we reach our forties, our fat starts to travel. In fact, about 50 percent of the fat that settles in our bellies is composed of fat that was once located elsewhere on our bodies. Once there, it turns from protective subcutaneous fat to dangerous visceral fat, meeting up with immune cells to create a vicious cycle of increased weight and inflammation.

Part of this shift has to do with lost muscle. One study found that men aged sixty to sixty-nine weigh an average of eight pounds more than their peers aged twenty to twenty-nine, but have fourteen pounds less muscle; older women weigh twelve pounds more than their younger counterparts despite having thirteen fewer pounds of muscle. But the primary driver is hormonal: As estrogen and testosterone drop, our protection against the growth of visceral fat drops as well.

As weight grows and muscle declines, our body reassesses its relationship with food and fat. When we are lean, about 5 percent of our glucose—the sugar in our blood that's formed from the calories we consume—is directed toward our fatty tissue, with the rest of it being used for energy or stored in our liver or muscles. But as we gain weight, this shifts; in obese individuals, about 20 percent of that glucose is directed right into the fat cells. Fat begets fat.

This is why building muscle is so important to keeping our bellies lean, our inflammation low, and our microbiome healthy.

HOW THE FULL-BODY FAT FIX PROTECTS LIFESAVING MUSCLE

Most weight-loss programs are, at their core, muscle-loss programs as well. In overweight or obese people, about 20 to 30 percent of the weight lost on a typical calorie-restriction diet is muscle.

The reason is simple: We evolved in a time of scarcity, when every meal involved a fight for survival, not just a quick car ride to Trader Joe's. So, when we cut calories to lose weight, our bodies would much prefer to give up calorie-burning muscle rather than calorie-hoarding fat. It's one reason why most weight-loss plans result in rebound weight gain; we sacrifice muscle, can't burn as many calories, can't store as much blood sugar, can't fight as effectively against inflammation. Once we stop restricting calories and go back to eating normally, the table is set for fat and inflammation to wreak even greater havoc.

That's why the Full-Body Fat Fix includes significant doses of protein at every meal, but especially at breakfast; protein has been shown to be a key nutrient for maintaining healthy muscle. One recent study at Wake Forest University looked at the effects of low- or high-protein diets. Those in the high-protein group not only lost more weight than the low-protein group, but a greater percentage of the weight loss was from fat; the protein helped participants hold on to their muscle mass while improving bone quality and decreasing their risk of numerous health issues, including diabetes and stroke. Combining diet with resistance training magnifies this result.

We've already explained how older bodies need larger doses of protein—between 25 and 30 grams at every meal, plus additional protein with each snack—to "pull the trigger" on the process of protein synthesis, the process by which we convert dietary protein into muscle. And we've shown how the average American eats just 10 grams of protein, on average, at breakfast—a diet plan that's perfectly designed to increase muscle loss as we get older.

But protein quantity is only part of the equation: Protein quality also matters. "Complete" proteins that include the entire range of amino acids do a far better job of stimulating muscle maintenance. In particular, the amino acid leucine—found in animal products, especially dairy, as well as soy protein—seems to be the strongest independent predictor of protein-muscle response.

When it comes to preserving muscle while you lose weight, protein alone won't do the trick. We may not think of fruits and vegetables as body builder fare, but they are. Indeed, a study in the *Journal of Nutrition* followed 3,759 people over the course of twelve years; at the end of the study, those who ate the most leafy greens were stronger, faster, and had more powerful legs than those who ate the least. So, as you pursue your goal of hitting thirty different plants in each week, you're doing more than just making your belly bugs happy. You're feeding your muscles as well. Consider what's on your plate:

- Fruits and vegetables: How would you like an additional 3.6 pounds of lean, healthy muscle? That's how much older people who ate lots of potassium-rich produce in one study had, compared to their peers who ate only half as much potassium. Think bananas, of course, but also broccoli, spinach, tomatoes, cantaloupe, dried apricots, and prunes. Researchers have also discovered an association between higher levels of dietary vitamin C intake and greater muscle mass—more reasons to enjoy citrus fruits as well as berries, bell peppers, kiwi, cauliflower, tomatoes, and the mighty broccoli. Keep it up and you'll see quick payoffs: One small study of older adults found that those who increased their fruit and vegetable intake from two portions a day to five portions a day showed greater grip strength after sixteen weeks.
- Beans and legumes: When the Cleveland Clinic polled dietitians about their most recommended sources of protein, Greek yogurt, eggs, and wild salmon were predictably in the top four. But their number one recommendation: beans, lentils, and split peas. Legumes provide protein and fiber; they even contain modest amounts of the crucial muscle-building amino acid leucine. And, like leafy greens, they're high in the B vitamin folate: In one study of older people with diabetes, the higher a person's folate levels, the greater their leg strength and grip strength.
- Nuts, seeds, and healthy oils: The type of fat in your diet impacts the type of fat in your muscles; opt for monounsaturated fats found in nuts, seeds, olives, and avocados, and it's like hitting the Tin Man with a healthy oil can, leading to healthier, better-functioning muscles. Nuts, seeds, avocado, and olives are also excellent sources of vitamin E, which, like other antioxidants, help to protect the health of bodily tissues. Since our muscles consume more oxygen than any other part of our bodies, they're more susceptible to damage caused by free radicals—those loose atoms or molecules that are the natural side effects of day-to-day living. But vitamin E (in food, not in pills) helps to prevent age-related damage to our muscles by, among other things, rounding up these rogue troublemakers. Another crucial nutrient healthy fats deliver: magnesium, which is found in high levels in pumpkin

seeds, almonds, cashews, and peanuts. One study found higher blood levels of magnesium were associated with stronger grip strength and leg-muscle power in older adults.

- Vitamin D–rich and calcium-rich dairy foods: Healthy vitamin D levels can help increase your muscular performance levels and reduce your risk of falls. Calcium also plays a major role in helping muscles function smoothly and contributes to a healthy blood pressure, as well as serving as the foundation of bone health: About 54 million Americans have osteoporosis or its precursor, osteopenia. How life-altering is low bone density? Studies suggest that approximately one in two women and as many as one in four men aged fifty and older will break a bone due to osteoporosis. The disease is responsible for an estimated two million broken bones per year. And breaking bones can be deadly: Nearly one in four hip fracture patients aged fifty and older die in the year following the fracture. Protecting your muscles is a crucial element of protecting your bones.

BEYOND DIET: IT'S TIME TO JOIN THE RESISTANCE

Eating a protein- and nutrient-rich diet is a critical aspect of protecting your muscle mass, but it's not enough. Strong, healthy muscles require exercise. Specifically, weight-bearing, or resistance, exercise— weight training, yoga, Pilates, calisthenics, and other workouts that challenge our muscles and help us stay strong.

If you're a runner, a biker, or just an avid dog walker, keep it up. Cardiovascular exercise helps to reduce weight gain and reduce your risk of heart disease by keeping the lungs and heart muscle strong and the arteries and veins clear of plaque buildup. But you need a complete workout plan, an exercise design that helps to convert fat into energy, reduces inflammation, boosts the health of your microbiome, and increases your muscle mass.

Fortunately, just such a workout exists. Simply turn to the next chapter, and let's get started!

Your Magic Muscles

Strongest: your jaw muscle, or masseter. The Guinness World Record for the strongest bite, set by a Florida man, was 975 pounds.

Fastest: the eyelid muscle, or orbicularis oculi. A blink of an eye, measured by researchers, lasts about 0.3 seconds.

Biggest: the butt muscle, or gluteus maximus. While we're back here, a tushy fat fact: Researchers suggest butt fat may boost cognitive performance because it tends to be higher in brain-boosting omega-3 fatty acids, while belly fat is higher in brain-inhibiting inflammatory compounds. Twerk it!

The Muscle Mufflers

It's not just inflammation. Here are four additional reasons we lose lean muscle as we age:

1. **Reduced physical activity.** We may work out less, eschewing the gym or the bike for less taxing activities. We may play less, giving up softball or skiing due to a bum knee or creaky shoulder. And we may walk less, drive more, and outsource tasks like mowing the lawn to neighborhood teenagers. All of these contribute to a reduction in the stress we put our muscles under.

2. **Elevated levels of free radicals.** These errant molecules are produced by your body whenever it breaks down food or manages toxins like tobacco smoke or pollution. Excessive free radicals accelerate the aging process on a cellular level, causing everything from wrinkles to heart disease to withering muscle. Certain vitamins, minerals, and other nutrients function as antioxidants, reducing the influence of free radicals.

3. **Mitochondrial dysfunction.** The mitochondria are the batteries that power our cells. As we age, our mitochondria function less effectively. There's a resulting give-and-take between mitochondria and muscle: As muscle declines, mitochondria appear

to become less efficient at generating energy, and vice versa. Think of a flashlight when the battery is running low. It may still function, but the light is dimmer.

4. **Hormonal changes.** Testosterone is one of the primary drivers of muscle maintenance, but its levels drop as we age. In men, testosterone dips about 1 percent per year after age thirty. Women also see a drop, particularly between the ages of twenty to forty-five. Other hormones, too, play a role in muscle maintenance: Estrogen, growth hormone, and vitamin D—technically a hormone, not a vitamin—also drop as we age.

10

The Best Exercise Plan for Your Gut

This scientifically proven workout program for your microbiome will help you burn fat, build muscle, and cut inflammation. Plus: A clever little cheat that will help you look slimmer, fast.

Have you ever imagined yourself as a championship athlete?

Let me put it another way: Have you ever imagined yourself as tens of trillions of tiny little championship athletes, all gathered in one body, with each one of you giving your all to win?

It turns out that the difference between Patrick Mahomes and the average football player might be more than just sheer talent and practice, practice, practice. It might have to do with the health of their gut bacteria. Studies show that elite athletes have a higher abundance of health-promoting bacteria and increased biodiversity in their microbiome. And those athletes in peak condition, with the highest levels of cardiovascular fitness, also have the highest levels of gut microbial diversity.

Will the time come when NFL scouts stop drafting players based on their 40-yard sprint times, and instead make their selections based on poop samples? We hope not. But research shows that the most physically fit, accomplished, and competitive humans are the ones who have the most physically fit belly bugs. When researchers compared elite rugby players with nonathletes who were otherwise lean and healthy, they found that the elite athletes averaged twice as many different strains of one type of bacteria as their less athletic counterparts. And research from the American Gut Project has found that

How a Post-Dinner Walk Can Change Your Gut—and Your Life

When we think about exercise, we often think about clanging metal in the gym, pounding the rubber of a treadmill, or pumping along to the provocations of a trainer on a video screen atop our Peloton bike.

But while we may think that a good workout requires sweating profusely or getting "shredded," "swole," "ripped," or whatever the lingo is today, when it comes to your microbiome, something far more modest may be just as important. In fact, the simple act of walking outdoors can be an especially effective form of exercise, especially when it comes to fighting inflammation, healing our guts, and giving our microbiomes a leg up.

Researchers recently conducted a review of seven studies and found that a light-intensity walk after a meal "significantly reduced postprandial glucose" levels, while sitting after a meal allowed blood glucose levels to rise unabated. Higher glucose levels mean a higher likelihood of weight gain, as the body is whammed with blood sugar and needs to find someplace to store it.

So simply taking a walk after every meal could have an enormous impact on your weight and overall health. But to maximize the health benefits, don't just tread around your living room. Get outside.

The more time you spend in the outdoors, the more diverse your microbiome can become. That's partly because you're exposing yourself to a wider variety of bacteria and yeast in the air, instead of just whatever's trapped in—or filtered out of—your office, living room, or local gym. Indeed, since the outbreak of the more frequently you exercise, the more diverse your microbiome becomes.

What kind of exercise? An extensive 2021 review of the link between exercise and gut health in *Frontiers in Nutrition* found that both moderate and intense exercise have positive effects on the gut

COVID-19, the market for air filters has exploded; a 2023 report by Grand View Research estimated that year's air-filtration market at $13.9 billion, but predicted the industry would nearly double to $26 billion by 2030.

But our attempt to protect ourselves from microbes in nature might very well undermine our body's ability to access something we badly need: those very same microbes found in nature. Because, along with a handful of nasty viruses, fungi, and allergens are untold trillions of microbes that work with our bodies in healthful ways.

"Get out in nature and get in contact with the microbes we evolved with," recommended Shilpa Ravella, MD, assistant professor of medicine at Columbia University Medical Center and author of *A Silent Fire*. "It could be getting out for a walk, or working in your garden. Mostly we are in our houses or offices, and if we exercise we are in gyms. A big part of the picture is being exposed to the right quantity and quality of germs."

Another way to boost your belly bugs is to go for a swim—not in the heavily chlorinated pool at the Y, but at a local lake or river or seashore. "When you think about your gut microbiome, well, that's just one piece," Ravella told me. "You have your skin microbiome, you have one in your lungs, and if you get some dirt on your feet or you wind up swallowing a bit of ocean water, your boundaries are expanding."

One Finnish study looked at children who played in the forest versus those who played in an urban daycare setting, and found that those who trekked through nature had more diverse microbiomes.

microbiome, but moderate exercise might be more effective at reducing inflammation and "leaky gut" and improving the mix of gut microbiota. Here's what the science tells us, and how to perform the ultimate workout for your gut health.

BUILDING A BUFF MICROBIOME

It's not yet clear why exercise has this powerful effect on our microbiome. One theory is that because exercise increases lactate in the body, it's possible that the resulting lactic acid helps feed these good-for-you bacteria. Another theory is that the increase in blood flow throughout the body might positively affect the cells of the gut wall. A third idea is that hormonal changes caused by exercise might give healthy bacteria a boost.

What we do know is that exercise increases the body's oxygen and energy demands. To help the body meet this need, the gut responds by boosting the number and diversity of species that produce short chain fatty acids (SCFAs), while potentially disease-causing species, such as E. coli, decrease.

And it doesn't take months, weeks, or even days of exercise to have this effect. In fact, you can improve the balance between the good guys and the bad guys in the course of a single exercise session: In one study, researchers took stool samples of twenty amateur athletes before and after they ran a half-marathon. They discovered that over the course of the race, the athletes' guts showed an increase in twenty healthy and diverse microbes.

Not ready for a half-marathon? Not a problem. Another study looked at sedentary people who had been diagnosed with diabetes or prediabetes. Half did high-intensity interval training; half did moderate-intensity, steady-state workouts. Both training methods increased levels of *Bacteroidetes,* a group of gut bacteria that helps the immune system to produce anti-inflammatory compounds. (Studies link high levels of these bacteria to a reduced risk of obesity.)

The key is to find an exercise intensity that works for you—one that you can stick with, because consistency is the key. One study found that when people began a cardio fitness plan, the quality of their gut microbiome changed dramatically after *just one week*, suggesting that the microbiome steps up quickly to answer the call and remains healthier throughout the exercise program. But the researchers also found that the positive changes rapidly diminished once the exercise period passed.

And you can mix it up as you see fit: Another study looked at thirty-two women who exercised at various intensities for six weeks; during that time they varied their exercise between thirty and sixty minutes at a time, and between 60 percent of their maximum heart rate (a pace at which you can talk comfortably and maintain breathing) to 75 percent, which is break-a-sweat territory. At the end of six weeks, the subjects showed great improvements in microbiome diversity. But then the subjects were instructed to stop exercising for six weeks. The result: By the end of the inactivity period, all the subjects' guts had returned to their original states, suggesting again that it's less the intensity or duration of your workout than your commitment to stick with it that counts.

The Pill That Kills Your Skills

Study after study has found that the fitter your microbiome, the higher your overall fitness level and the better your potential athletic performance. Yet elite athletes take antibiotics twice as often as the average person, in a misguided effort to stave off illnesses that could cut down on their ability to compete.

Lately, researchers have linked the overuse of antibiotics—which can be devastating to the microbiome—to muscle weakness, pain, and even a reduced competitive spirit. In animal studies, mice that had been bred to be elite runners were slower and less motivated to exercise after a course of antibiotics. The journal *Sports Health* even issued a warning to "athletes of all ages" that routine antibiotics use has been linked to a number of sports injuries, as well as "decreased performance."

THE BEST-EVER BELLY-BUG WORKOUT

I've created a fitness program based on studies of the human microbiome, which consistently show that a combination of moderate aerobic exercise and resistance training is an effective way to boost diversity in your gut, with implications for improved heart health, a more effective immune system, and a healthier and sharper brain.

As long as you're following the Full-Body Fat Fix, and starting each day with 30 grams of protein, you'll maximize the efficacy of this plan. In studies, those who followed this workout and supplemented with 30 grams of whey protein per day showed lower weight, lower body fat percentage, and improved gut microbiome after eight weeks. You'll be amazed how quickly you can . . .

- Trim inches off your belly
- Burn unwanted fat
- Build lean, strong, toned muscle
- Improve your insulin sensitivity
- Lower your blood pressure and protect your heart
- Feel stronger, more mobile, and more energetic

Warm-up: Five-minute easy jog or brisk walk on treadmill, or light warm-up on another machine.

Cardio portion: Moderate-intensity aerobic workout for eighteen minutes on the cardio machine of your choice. Over the course of the next eight weeks, look to work up to thirty-two minutes. You can vary between rowing, biking, stairclimbing, running, or walking briskly. Aim for an intensity level that allows you to still hold a conversation, even if you're breathing just a little heavier.

Resistance exercise portion: Pick three upper body exercises, three lower body exercises, and one core exercise from the list that follows. Feel free to vary these exercises to keep it interesting.

Start with a weight you can lift for three sets of eight reps, with the last set being challenging. (Typically, about 50 to 70 percent of your one-rep max.) As you get stronger, increase the number of reps in each set. Once you can do three sets of twelve reps comfortably and with correct form, increase the weight, drop back down to eight reps, and start again. Look to increase weight by 15 to 20 percent over the course of eight weeks. In a 2023 study at the University of Missouri-Columbia, those who followed this program showed lower fasting glucose, lower blood pressure, and lower waist circumference. They also showed significant increases in specific bacteria that are known to protect against weight gain and insulin resistance.

Stretches: Do the **flat-belly stretch** (directions on page 177) and at least one additional stretch at each workout. I've given you an array of stretches for your lower body, but make sure you take advantage of one of the easiest and most effective flat-belly hacks ever.

As our bellies get bigger, our hips begin to tilt forward, giving us a hunched-over appearance and making us look older and heavier than we are. Compounding this is the amount of time we spend in a seated position: The more hours we spend with our knees close to our bellies, the more our hip flexors—the muscles that run down the front of our hips and help us lift our legs—become shorter and tighter. But the flat-belly stretch can correct this pelvic tilt and help you cheat your way to a leaner look.

UPPER BODY EXERCISES

Pick one exercise from each row
Chest / Shoulders / Back
1. Chest press / Overhead press / Upright row
2. Incline chest press / Lateral side raise / Seated row
3. Decline pushups or dips / Alternating front raise / Face pull
4. Flies / Bent-over reverse flies / One-arm dumbbell row

LOWER BODY EXERCISES

Pick any three
Squat
Sumo deadlift
Weighted step-up

Hamstring curl
Kickback
Leg press

CORE EXERCISES

Pick one
Farmer's walk (dumbbell in one hand)
Plank
Side plank
Crunch
Leg lift

STRETCHES

At every workout
Flat-belly stretch

Plus, add at least one of the following
Standing quadriceps stretch
Hip and thigh stretch
Iliotibial band stretch
Lying figure four

HOW TO DO THEM

Note: The best setting for this workout is a gym. That will allow you to switch off between machines and free weights as you see fit, and to increase your weights as you get stronger. (See How to Find [and Use] the Best Gym, page 179.) But to get you started, I've included descriptions for how you can do the entire workout at home. All you need is an exercise mat, one or two yoga blocks or towels, a firm resistance band, and some hand weights.

CHEST

Pick one

Chest Press: Grab a weight in each hand and lie on your back on an exercise bench. Bend your legs and plant your feet on the floor.

Hold the weights above your shoulders, with your elbows bent. Now straighten your arms, pushing the weights into the air above you. Don't lock your elbows. At the top, pause for a moment and then bend your elbows to slowly lower the weights down as close to your chest as you can.

At-home option: Place a folded towel or yoga block on an exercise mat and lie back on the mat so your upper back rests on the block or towel. (The idea here is to create enough space between your body and the floor that you can lower the weights to your chest.) Follow the instructions above.

Incline Chest Press: Grab a weight in each hand and lie on your back on an exercise bench inclined to about 30 degrees. Bend your legs and plant your feet on the floor. Hold the weights above your shoulders, with your elbows bent. Now straighten your arms, pushing the weights into the air above you. Don't lock your elbows. At the top, pause for a moment and then bend your elbows to slowly lower the weights down as close to your chest as you can.

At-home option: Place two or three folded towels or two yoga blocks on an exercise mat and lie back on the mat so your upper back rests on the blocks or towels. (Your upper body should be at about a 30-degree angle.) Follow the instructions above.

Decline Pushups: This is a slightly more challenging version of a standard pushup; if it feels too challenging, feel free to start with a standard pushup (toes on the floor) or even a kneeling pushup. Place a yoga block or similar-sized, sturdy object on one end of an exercise mat. Lie face down on the mat with your feet on the object or block. Place your hands directly below your shoulders, palms flat on the mat, elbows bent and tucked in at your sides. Engage your core. Now, keeping your back straight, push up with your hands until your arms are fully extended. Don't lock your elbows. Pause for a moment, then lower back down.

Dips: Place a chair with its back against a wall for stability. Sit on the chair, place your hands near your hips, and grasp the chair seat with each hand. Supporting your weight on your hands, lift your butt off the chair and scoot your legs out in front of you until they are almost straight, feet flat on the floor. Keeping your shoulders back, chin up, and neck straight, bend your elbows and slowly lower your body toward the floor until your elbows are bent at a 45-degree angle. Pause for a moment, then straighten your elbows as you push yourself upward. Don't thrust your hips; keep your lower body relaxed but straight so all the effort comes from your arms, chest, and shoulders. (If this feels too hard to start, bring your feet closer to the chair and keep your knees bent to reduce the amount of weight your arms have to bear.)

Flies: Grab a weight in each hand and lie back on an exercise bench inclined to about 30 degrees. Bend your legs and plant your feet on the floor. Hold the weights above your shoulders, with your elbows bent. Push the weights up until your arms are straight and turn your palms to face each other. This is the starting position. Now bend your elbows as you slowly bring the weights down in a wide arc; imagine you're trying to broaden your chest. Lower the weights to where they are even with your chest. Pause for a moment, then use your chest and arm muscles to push the weights back to the starting position.

At-home option: Place two or three folded towels or two yoga blocks on an exercise mat. Grab a weight in each hand and lie back on the mat so your upper back rests on the blocks or towels. (Your upper body should be at about a 30-degree angle.) Follow the instructions above.

SHOULDERS

Pick one

Overhead Press: Stand with your back straight, feet flat on the floor, knees slightly bent. Hold a light weight in each hand. Bend and lift your elbows so your upper arms are parallel to the floor, elbows at 90 degrees, your hands by your ears, palms facing out. Now press your arms up into the air over your head; try to extend your arms fully and touch your hands over your head. Pause for a moment, then lower the weights.

Lateral Side Raise: Stand with your feet shoulder-width apart and hold a weight in each hand. Bring the weights together in front of your hips, palms facing each other. Tilt slightly forward at the hips for balance. Now, keeping your lower body still, bring your arms up and out like a bird taking flight. Always keep a slight bend in your elbows to prevent putting too much strain on the tendons in your shoulders. At the top of the motion, your hands should be even with or just slightly above your shoulders. Pause for a moment, then lower back down until your arms are almost, but not quite, perpendicular to the ground. (Keep your movements smooth. If you feel the need to shrug or jerk the weights to lift them up, you're using too much weight.)

Alternating Front Raise: Stand with your feet shoulder-width apart and hold a weight in each hand, with your hands at the sides of your hips, palms facing in. Brace your legs, hips, and core so you are solidly anchored in place. Lift your left arm straight out in front of you until the weights are at eye level, turning your wrist so that your palm faces the floor at the top of the motion. Pause for a moment, then return to the starting position. Repeat the movement with your right arm. (Keep your movements smooth. If you feel the need to shrug or jerk the weights to lift them up, you're using too much weight.)

Bent-Over Reverse Flies: Stand with your feet shoulder-width apart and hold a weight in each hand. Bring the weights together in front of your hips, palms facing your thighs. Bend forward at the hips at about a 60-degree angle. Keep your chin up, neck straight, eyes on the floor in front of you. Lift the weights up and back; at the top of the movement the weights should be slightly behind you at shoulder level, and your palms should be facing the wall behind you. Pause for a moment, then lower the weights. (Keep your movements smooth. If you feel the need to shrug or jerk the weights to lift them up, you're using too much weight.)

BACK

Pick one

Upright Row: Stand with your feet shoulder-width apart and hold a weight in each hand, with your hands in front of you and your palms facing your thighs. Keeping the weights close to the front of your body, bend your elbows up and out, lifting the weights up the front of your body until they are just in front of your shoulders. Squeeze your shoulder blades together at the top of the movement. Pause for a moment, then return to the starting position.

Seated Row: Wrap an exercise band around something very sturdy, like a support beam. Place a mat in front of the beam and sit down facing it. Brace your feet against the beam with your legs straight, knees slightly bent. Grab one end of the band in each hand. Sit with your back straight, chin up, eyes forward, arms extended forward, palms facing one another. Keeping your back, legs, and hips still, use the muscles of your middle back and arms to pull your elbows back until your hands are at your hips. Try to touch your shoulder blades together at the top of the movement. Pause for a moment, then return to the starting position.

Face Pull: While it sounds like a painful maneuver used in pro wrestling, this move is actually a gentle and effective exercise for the upper back. Sit on a mat with your legs straight and wrap an exercise band around the middle of your soles (not your toes). Grasp one end of the band in each hand, with your palms facing the floor, and slide your hands up the band until you're holding it firm against your feet. Now bend your elbows out to the sides, as though you were riding a motorcycle. This is the starting position. Keeping your legs and torso still and your elbows wide, pull your shoulders and elbows back until your hands are at the sides of your ears. Try to touch your shoulder blades together at the top of the movement. Pause for a moment, then return to the starting position.

One-Arm Dumbbell Row: Place a chair with its back against a wall for stability. Stand facing the chair, feet shoulder-width apart. Hold a weight in your right hand. Bend forward at the waist with a flat back (your back should be parallel to the ground) and place your left hand, arm extended, on the seat of the chair for support. Keeping your back parallel to the ground, allow your right arm to extend toward the floor while your right hand is holding the weight. Your palm should be facing your body. Now, keeping your right arm close to your side, bend your right elbow, using the muscles of your upper back to pull the weight up until it's next to your rib cage. Slowly lower the weight back to the starting position. After eight reps, switch the weight to your left hand and perform the exercise on your left side.

LEGS

Pick three

Squat: Stand with your feet shoulder-width apart, feet flat on the floor. Hold a weight to your chest with both hands. Now slowly bend your knees and lower your butt as if you were sitting on a chair. When your thighs are parallel to the floor, stop, pause for a moment, and then use your core, glutes, hamstrings, and quads to stand back up a bit more quickly than you squatted down.

Don't squat below parallel or let your knees drift out in front of your toes or inward toward the midline of your body, which can put you at risk for knee problems.

Sumo Deadlift: Stand with your feet slightly wider than shoulder-width apart, feet flat on the floor, toes pointed slightly outward. Rest two weights on the floor between your legs. Keeping your back straight, chest back, chin up, eyes forward, bend your knees and lower your butt toward the floor until you can grab a weight in each hand. Tilt back gently to lift the weights slightly off the floor, keeping your arms hanging straight down throughout the exercise. Now use your core, glutes, hamstrings, and quads to stand up.

Don't let your knees drift inward toward the midline of your body, which can put you at risk for knee problems.

Weighted Step-Up: Stand at the bottom of a staircase, holding the railing with your right hand for support. (You can also use a stable platform, if you don't need a railing for support.) With your left hand, hold a weight, allowing it to hang down at thigh level. Now step with your left leg onto the bottom stair and lift your body up as you bend your right leg comfortably behind you. Pause for a moment, then lower your right leg to the floor and return to the starting position. Switch the weight to your right hand and repeat the movement, this time stepping up with your right leg, keeping your left leg behind you, and using your left hand to hold the railing for support. Pause for a moment, then return to the starting position.

Hamstring Curl: Hamstring curl machines are available in most gyms, but you can get the same effect at home using a dumbbell. Place the dumbbell on its end on one end of a mat. Lie face down on the mat with the dumbbell between your feet. Support your head with your hands. Now, use the soles of your feet to hold onto the end of the dumbbell and slowly bend both knees as you bring the dumbbell up toward your butt. Pause at the top of the movement, then slowly lower the weight.

Kickback: Kickback machines are available in most gyms and are terrific for working your butt muscles—the largest muscles in the body, and hence the ones that give you the most bang for your buck. To duplicate the effects without a machine, place a chair with its back against the wall for stability. Grab a light dumbbell in your right hand. Stand in front of the chair with your feet slightly less than shoulder-width apart, so you can comfortably bend forward and rest your left hand on the seat of the chair. Place the dumbbell behind your right knee and bend the knee 90 degrees to lock the dumbbell in place. Place your right hand on the seat of the chair, so that you're now holding on to the chair with both hands. Keeping your right knee bent to hold the dumbbell in place, engage your right glute, and slowly kick your right leg back behind you. At the top of the motion, your right thigh should be parallel to the ground, with the bottom of your right foot elevated toward the ceiling. Pause for a moment and lower your leg. When finished with the set, switch the dumbbell to your left leg and repeat.

Leg Press: Found in almost every commercial gym, leg press machines are a safe and effective alternative to squats. To replicate the exercise without the machine, grab a thick exercise band. Lie on your back on a mat, and hold one end of the exercise band in each hand. Wrap the middle of the band around the soles of your feet. Bring your knees to your chest, and work your hands up the band until it is tight around your feet. Place your upper arms on the mat and bend your elbows 90 degrees, palms facing the sides of your body. Now, extend your legs straight out and upward; at the top of the motion your hips should form about a 45-degree angle with the floor. Do not lock your knees. Pause for a moment, then bend your knees and bring them back to your chest. As you get stronger, you can increase the resistance by grabbing the band closer to your feet.

CORE

Pick one

Farmer's Walk: Brace your abdominal muscles, and pick up a weight in your right hand. Stand with your arms straight down at your sides, palms facing your hips. Stand tall and straight: Pull your shoulders back, and imagine a string at the very top of your head pulling you toward the ceiling. Now, keeping the weight at your side, walk for fifteen seconds. You'll feel the muscles on the left side of your torso working to keep you erect. After fifteen seconds, stop, gently place the weight on the ground, then pick it up with your left hand, and repeat the exercise for fifteen seconds to work the right side of your torso.

Plank: Lie face down, legs straight, toes touching the floor. Bend your arms at the elbow and rest your forearms on the floor below you. Now, keeping your neck and back straight, lift your hips and chest off the floor, so your weight is resting on your forearms and toes. Hold for three breaths—or more, as you grow stronger—then lower yourself back to the floor.

Side Plank: Lie on your right side on a mat, and support your weight on your right elbow, which should be directly below your shoulder. Cross your left foot over your right so both are resting on the mat. Engage your core, then lift your hips into the air to form a straight line from your shoulder down to your ankles. Hold this position for three breaths—or more, as you grow stronger—then lower yourself back to the floor.

Crunch: Lie on a mat on your back, knees bent, feet flat on the floor. Cross your hands over your chest. Keeping your neck straight (don't look down), slowly curl your shoulders off the floor and toward your knees as far as you can. At the top of the movement, pause, and then slowly lower back down.

Leg Lift: Lie on your back on a mat with your legs flat on the mat. Slide your hands underneath your hips, so that the hip bones are cushioned by the fatty part of your hand, between your thumb and forefinger. Now engage your core and, keeping your legs straight, raise your legs an inch or two off the ground. Hold for one second, then spread your legs gently, keeping them suspended above the floor, and hold for one second. Then bring your legs together, and hold for one second. Now lower your legs to the floor.

STRETCHES

Do this at every workout

Flat-Belly (or Hip Flexor) Stretch: Place your left knee on a mat, with your right knee bent at 90 degrees, right foot flat on the mat. Reach your left hand up over your head toward your right shoulder and, as you do so, engage your butt muscles. Now lean farther to the right as you push forward with your left knee. You should feel a stretch in your left hip flexor, the muscle that runs down the front of your left hip. Hold the stretch for eight long breaths, then relax and switch sides to stretch the right hip flexor. Repeat on each side three to four times at the end of every workout. As you become more comfortable, extend the length of each stretch to about twelve breaths.

Add one of the following at every workout

Standing Quadriceps Stretch: Stand about a foot away from a wall, facing the wall. Rest your left arm against the wall for balance. Bend your right knee and lift your right foot up behind you, so your lower leg is about parallel with the floor. Now, with your right hand, reach down and grab your right foot. Gently pull upward on the foot so you feel a light stretch in the front of your right thigh. Hold for thirty to sixty seconds, then gently release your foot and lower it to the ground. Repeat with your left leg. Relax and repeat.

Hip and Thigh Stretch: Stand tall with your feet wider than shoulder-width apart. Turn your feet, hips, and shoulders to the right. Now bend your right leg and lower your body so that your right thigh is parallel with the ground and your right calf is perpendicular to the ground. Lower your body as much as you feel comfortable, until you feel a stretch in the muscles on the inside of your right thigh. Hold for thirty to sixty seconds, then straighten back up to the starting position. Repeat the motion to the left side. Relax and repeat.

Iliotibial Band Stretch: Did you know your body comes with its own band? Two of them, actually, called the iliotibial bands (ITB). The ITB is a thick band of tissue that runs down the outside of each of your thighs, connecting your hips to your knees. When the ITB gets tight, it can cause hip pain, knee pain, or both. To stretch the ITB, sit on the floor with your legs stretched out in front of you and your back straight. Place your hands on the floor next to you for balance. Bend your right knee and place your right foot on the floor on the outside of your left knee. Turn your head and shoulders so you are facing toward the right. Lift your left arm and place it against the outside of your right knee. Now gently press your left arm against your right knee, pushing it farther across your body; you should feel a stretch along the right side of your hip and spine. Hold for thirty to sixty seconds, then repeat on the opposite side.

Lying Figure Four: Lie on your back with your knees bent. Cross your right ankle over your left knee and rest it there. Now reach both hands down and grasp the back of your left leg just below the knee. Gently pull your left leg toward you, being sure to keep your upper body flat against the floor. Hold for thirty to sixty seconds. Repeat on the opposite side.

How to Find (and Use) the Best Gym

People with gym memberships are fourteen times more aerobically active than nonmembers and ten times more likely to meet muscle-strengthening guidelines, according to a 2017 study—and that's true even if they've been members for less than a year.

And you don't need to spend a fortune to join. Maybe you don't mind paying extra for a glass-enclosed health club with tanning pods and a juice bar. But a basic membership at a local gym or YMCA will give you access to everything you need for a great workout, and you don't need to pay a premium to have a masseuse spritz you with rose water.

If you're looking for a gym, be sure to visit during the hours you'd actually want to attend. Ninety-one percent of people who have gym memberships are between the ages of eighteen and fifty-four. That means most gyms are slammed before and right after work, and at lunchtime. If you have the flexibility to go at, say, 3 P.M., you might find you have the place practically to yourself. That said, many Ys cater to students and seniors, so you may find the flow of the crowd to be different in those locations.

Make sure the gym you choose has an array of free weights as well as exercise machines. While you may use machines for some of these exercises, there are several reasons to choose free weights. First, free weights allow you to move through a range of motion that's unique to your body, rather than locking you in to a motion prescribed by a machine. Delicate joints like the shoulders and knees are less likely to be injured. Second, free weights make it harder for you to cheat—using the stronger limb to help out the weaker one—yet another way that machines set you up for injury.

Finally, the gym is really a hall of mirrors, one that amplifies both our attributes and shortcomings. Because feeling good starts with looking good, there's nothing wrong with investing in some flattering gym clothes you feel confident in. Think solid, dark colors that match top to bottom but cut to show off the parts you like. A worn-out gray T-shirt against pale winter skin can make you feel less like a powerful athlete in training and more like you're slogging through the gulag.

11

The Fat Fix Recipes

*Fifteen ways to unleash the Power Plants
(and fats and proteins) that will tickle even
the most trepidatious of taste buds.*

Every October, without fail, I pull out my torn, stained, crusty-in-places copy of *The Joy of Cooking*, open it to the page on pies, and begin making my favorite pumpkin pie recipe from scratch.

I've been pulling recipes, tips, and kitchen hacks from this book since I got a copy of it for my first wedding. I'm now twenty years into my *second* marriage, which gives you an idea of how long I've been opening the same book and cooking the same pie recipe.

Yes, I could Google a pumpkin pie recipe on my smartphone; you can Google pretty much any recipe nowadays. But most recipe sites make it impossible to follow their instructions, between the popup ads and the subscription solicitations and the phone constantly powering down if you're not continuously scrolling. Plus, because the sites want you to stay on the page for as long as possible, you'll inevitably have to scroll through paragraph after paragraph about how this old family recipe was smuggled past the Cossacks and out of the Old Country in the author's grandmother's babushka, or some other emotional family story designed to keep you lingering forever, when all you really want is a list of spices you need for your batter.

That's not going to happen here. My paternal grandmother, Rose, held a Depression-era approach to cooking that typically involved opening a can of green beans and boiling them in water until they reached the approximate consistency of a mud mask. My maternal grandmother, Eleanor, bequeathed us no family recipes but did once threaten to gouge out a man's eyeball with a hat pin. So, for me, learning to cook has meant starting at zero. Which is why all the recipes in this book will be exceedingly simple, yet packed with plenty of plant power! (And a minimal amount of annoying family lore!)

What matters most in these recipes is plant diversity. So, if you have no time for shopping, do some swapping: Make sure each meal has at least four unique Power Plants, and substitute them at will. These recipes aren't meant to be Talmudic; instead, they're a rough guide to getting as many diverse Power Plants into your diet as possible.

Sneaky Salmon "Salad"

NUMBER OF POWER PLANTS: 5+

SERVES 2–3

Everyone loves salmon. Even people who don't like fish like salmon. Which makes it the perfect delivery system for a wide range of plants. This dish doesn't look or taste like a salad, but in many ways that's just what it is: a bouquet of inflammation-busting plants on a platter of yummy orange meat. Consider serving with quinoa and a side salad for even more plant power.

INGREDIENTS

1 salmon fillet (about 1 pound)

1 tablespoon extra-virgin olive oil

1 teaspoon garlic powder

Sea salt and pepper to taste

Fresh sprigs of thyme, rosemary, parsley, sage, whatever

1 cup roasted red peppers, cut into thin strips

1 cup precooked, quartered artichoke hearts in olive oil

½ dozen fresh cherry tomatoes, halved

1 dozen kalamata olives, pitted and halved

DIRECTIONS

1. Preheat the oven to 325°F.
2. Lay salmon skin side down on a baking sheet. Drizzle on the olive oil, and sprinkle with garlic powder, salt, and pepper.
3. Strip the leaves from about half of the fresh herb sprigs and chop finely. Sprinkle the chopped leaves over the salmon.*
4. Scatter peppers, artichokes, tomatoes, and olives on top of the salmon.
5. Top with the remaining herb sprigs.
6. Bake the salmon in oven for 25 minutes or until just cooked through.

*By chopping the herbs you'll ensure that you actually eat them, upping your total plant intake. The more various herbs you add, the closer you get to your goal of thirty different plants!

The numbers: 285 calories; 5 g fiber; 25 g protein; 1 g sugar (0 added)

Tom's Big Game Day Chili

NUMBER OF POWER PLANTS: 5

SERVES 7–10

Buying fresh peppers is a great way to introduce a child to the whole notion of diversity, both in plants and in life—an idea I picked up from my dad, Tom. While we may have preconceived notions of what a pepper is (round, green, and bland), peppers are, in fact, like people: They come in all different shapes, colors, sizes, and intensity levels. I like red and yellow bell peppers, because they are higher in vitamin content than green peppers and hold their vibrant colors best in the chili mix. (Orange peppers, while beautiful at first, seem to blend in and get lost in the melting pot.) Low-intensity bell peppers allow you to add heat to taste; I have been burned (literally) by experimenting with habaneros or Scotch bonnets.

INGREDIENTS

   1–2 medium yellow onions, peeled
   1 large red bell pepper
   1 large yellow bell pepper
   1 tablespoon extra-virgin olive oil
   1½ pounds grass-fed ground beef, buffalo, turkey, or
       venison
   Salt, pepper, chili powder, and hot sauce, to taste
   2 (16-ounce) cans whole, peeled tomatoes
   1 small child
   1 (16-ounce) can dark red kidney beans
   1 (16-ounce) can black beans
   1 cup cooked brown rice (for vegan option) per serving

DIRECTIONS

1. Dice onions. Seed and dice peppers, discarding seeds and ribs.

2. In a large skillet, heat the olive oil. Add the peppers and onion and cook until slightly softened (2 to 3 minutes).

3. Shred the beef by hand and add to the skillet, stirring occasionally until fully browned (3 to 5 minutes). At this point, you may want to add a dash of salt, some black pepper, and chili powder, to infuse the meat. Go easy on the salt (but not on the chili powder!). When the meat is fully browned, remove meat and vegetable mixture from heat and set aside.

4. Now the fun part: Empty the cans of whole tomatoes into a large pot. Place a small child with clean hands on a step stool by the kitchen counter. Have him or her reach into the pot and mush the tomatoes by hand until they reach a stringy, soupy consistency (the tomatoes, not the hands).

5. Add the beans, including the liquid. (The liquid contains additional fiber and nutrients.)

6. Stir in the meat, peppers, and onions.

7. Simmer the mixture over low heat for 1½ hours, adding salt, pepper, chili powder, and hot sauce to taste. Do not be stingy

with the chili powder—contrary to what people often think, chili powder adds a smoky flavor, not a spicy one.

Make it vegan: Eliminate the meat and serve over cooked brown rice to create a complete protein profile.

The numbers: 365 calories; 10 g fiber; 31 g protein; 6 g sugar (0 added)

No More Sufferin' Succotash

NUMBER OF POWER PLANTS: 5

SERVES 3 (AS A SIDE DISH)

This recipe replaces the traditional lima beans with edamame, because . . . lima beans. It also pumps up the plant power with a wider array of vegetables, and will sit nicely with a piece of chicken or fish.

INGREDIENTS

1 tablespoon extra-virgin olive oil

½ onion, peeled and diced

1 red bell pepper, seeded and diced

1¼ cups precooked and shelled edamame, thawed if frozen

1¼ cups frozen corn kernels, thawed

½ cup grilled, frozen asparagus, thawed and chopped

1 teaspoon paprika

½ teaspoon garlic salt

¼ teaspoon coarsely ground black pepper

6 slices bacon, cooked, drained, and chopped

Sprigs of fresh thyme (or ½ teaspoon dried thyme)

DIRECTIONS

1. Heat the oil in a large pan over medium heat.

2. Add onion and bell pepper and cook, stirring, until tender (about 7 minutes).

3. Stir in edamame, corn, asparagus, paprika, garlic salt, black pepper, and bacon.

4. Hold the sprigs of thyme over the pan and carefully run your fingers down them, stripping the leaves off into pan. Discard stems.

5. Stir and reduce heat to low. Cover and simmer 3 to 5 minutes until warmed through.

Make it vegan: Replace the bacon with tempeh or seitan, and finish with an additional teaspoon of extra-virgin olive oil.

Note: For a creamy version, add ½ cup heavy cream and stir to coat vegetables before covering.

The numbers: 132 calories; 5.5 g fiber; 9 g protein; 5.5 g sugar (0 added)

Steak Sandwich with Aioli

NUMBER OF POWER PLANTS: 6+

SERVES 1

What to do with leftover steak? Slice it thinly and turn it into the most powerfully nutritional sandwich on the block.

INGREDIENTS

½ small precooked (leftover) ribeye or strip steak

1 portobello mushroom

1 tablespoon extra-virgin olive oil

Pinch salt

1 multigrain hoagie roll, sliced

¼ cup Dill Aioli (see recipe on page 187)

¼ cup kalamata olives, pitted and chopped

1 slice roasted red bell pepper (from jar)

1 small red onion, peeled and thinly sliced

Handful mesclun greens

DIRECTIONS

1. Remove leftover steak from fridge, slice thinly, and allow to reach room temperature (or briefly roast the slices, if you prefer).
2. Preheat the oven to 325°F.
3. Rub portobello with extra-virgin olive oil, place on a baking sheet, and season with salt. Roast for 12 to 15 minutes, until tender.
4. Lightly toast the hoagie roll in a toaster.
5. Smear one slice of the roll with aioli and spread the other with chopped olives.
6. Add steak slices, portobello, roasted pepper, red onion slices, and mesclun greens.

The numbers (includes aioli): 815 calories; 5 g fiber; 45 g protein; 9 g sugar (3 added)

DILL AIOLI

2 egg yolks
1 tablespoon Dijon mustard
¼ cup white wine vinegar
1 teaspoon sugar
¼ cup chopped dill
2 cups avocado oil

Mix all ingredients except for the oil in a bowl and whisk continuously. As you do, slowly stream in the oil until a thick mayonnaise forms. (You can also do this in a food processor or blender.) Store leftover aioli in an airtight container in the fridge for up to one week.

Totally Tubular Pasta with Grilled Chicken

NUMBER OF POWER PLANTS: 8

SERVES 3–4

Most of the time we eat pasta with just some meat and red sauce. That's fine, but here's a way to turn this natural crowd-pleaser into a Power Plant delivery system.

INGREDIENTS

1 box bucatini (or linguini) pasta
Pinch salt
1 cup extra-virgin olive oil
1 Vidalia onion, peeled and chopped
3 garlic cloves, peeled and chopped
6 shiitake mushrooms, stems removed and cut into ¼-inch strips
1 small graffiti eggplant, trimmed and cut into ¼-inch dice
1 small zucchini, halved lengthwise and cut into ¼-inch half moons
1 tablespoon finely chopped rosemary
2 cups precooked chicken, torn into small pieces
1 small Thai bird's eye chili, finely chopped (can substitute ½ jalapeño)
¼ cup finely chopped chives
¼ cup toasted breadcrumbs

DIRECTIONS

1. Boil pasta in lightly salted water, according to package instructions; drain and reserve ½ cup of the starchy pasta water.
2. In a sauté pan, heat olive oil and sweat onion and garlic over medium heat until softened and translucent.
3. Add mushrooms and sauté until soft and any water in the pan has cooked off.
4. Add eggplant and sauté until tender.

5. Add zucchini, rosemary, chicken, and half the chili (only start with half because these peppers can get *very* hot; taste and adjust to your preferences. You can always add, but you can't subtract).

6. Add your cooked pasta and some of the reserved pasta water, and toss until a sauce forms. Add chives, toss again, and plate topped with toasted breadcrumbs.

The numbers: 663 calories; 6 g fiber; 25 g protein; 3 g sugar (0 added)

Perfect Pizza

NUMBER OF POWER PLANTS: 5

SERVES 8 (4 SMALL PIZZAS)

If you'd like, you can start with a premade pizza crust like Boboli, and simply follow the baking instructions on the label. Or take it to another level and use a commercially available cauliflower crust. But making a pie totally from scratch marks you as the type of home cook who doesn't settle for whatever the delivery boy dragged in. And it's far easier than you might think.

INGREDIENTS (BASIC PIZZA DOUGH)

4 cups all-purpose flour (plus more for dusting)
1 packet (7 g) dry active yeast
Pinch salt
1½ cups warm water
2 tablespoons honey (optional, but if Wolfgang Puck does it, you probably should too)

INGREDIENTS (TOPPINGS)

4 cups crushed San Marzano tomatoes
4 cups fresh mozzarella, sliced
1 cup basil leaves, torn
½ cup fresh oregano leaves
4 black Mission figs, sliced
Handful arugula
8 strips thinly sliced prosciutto, chopped

DIRECTIONS

1. Mix flour, yeast, and salt together in a large bowl.
2. Add water and honey, then mix until a shaggy dough forms.
3. Empty dough onto a clean countertop and knead until a smooth, elastic dough forms (a stand mixer with a dough hook is good for this, if you have one).
4. Place in a lightly oiled bowl and cover with plastic wrap or a moist towel and let stand for 1 hour or until doubled in size.
5. Divide into four equal dough balls, place on a clean surface, and allow to stand a second time until doubled in size. (Each dough ball will make one small pizza; refrigerate extra dough balls for up to one week or freeze for up to three months.)
6. Preheat the oven to 400°F.
7. Coat a cold, 12-inch cast-iron skillet with extra-virgin olive oil. Place one dough ball into the pan and shape it so that it covers the bottom of the pan.
8. Cover the dough with one-fourth of the crushed tomatoes, mozzarella, basil, oregano, and figs.
9. Repeat steps 7 and 8 for each individual pizza (depending on how many skillets you have available). Make sure to use oven-safe skillets!
10. Heat the skillet(s) over medium heat until crust is sizzling and golden on the bottom.
11. Transfer the skillet(s) to the oven and cook until cheese is melted and begins to brown slightly.
12. Remove from the oven, top with arugula and prosciutto, and serve.

The numbers (per ½ pizza): 525 calories; 5 g fiber; 27.5 g protein; 14 g sugar (4 added)

Totally Lentil Soup

NUMBER OF POWER PLANTS: 7

SERVES 4

A terrific appetizer, this soup guarantees a plethora of Power Plants and all the fiber your microbiome could ask for.

INGREDIENTS

½ cup extra-virgin olive oil

1 medium carrot, peeled and cut into ¼-inch dice

1 sweet potato, peeled and cut into ¼-inch cubes

1 large leek, halved, cleaned, and sliced

1 medium bulb fennel, cored and cut into ¼-inch cubes

6 Sun Gold or yellow cherry tomatoes, halved

1 pound dried lentils

2 quarts vegetable stock

6 sprigs fresh thyme

4 ounces fresh spinach leaves

Salt, pepper, and lemon juice to taste

DIRECTIONS

1. In a large pot, add olive oil, carrot, sweet potato, leek, and fennel. Sweat the vegetables over medium-high heat until they are softened and the edges begin to take on a bit of color.

2. Add tomatoes and cook until the tomatoes have begun to break down and the water content has begun to evaporate.

3. When the pot begins to look a little dry, and some caramelization has occurred on the bottom of the pot, add in the dried lentils, stock, and thyme. Stir to make sure everything is evenly mixed and to scrape the caramelized bits off the bottom and bring to a simmer (not a boil).

4. Reduce the heat to low, and cook for 35 to 45 minutes, until the lentils are tender.

5. Add the fresh spinach, stirring just to wilt it a bit. Season with salt, pepper, and lemon juice to taste.

6. Remove the soup from heat and let sit for 10 to 15 minutes so the lentils absorb the seasoned broth. Taste and readjust the seasoning as needed. (Beans and lentils have a tendency to absorb the seasoning of the liquid around them, which can leave the soup seeming bland if you don't readjust the seasoning before serving. Since this recipe will give you plenty of extra soup, it's worthwhile to check the seasoning each time before you serve leftovers.)

The numbers: 424 calories; 12 g fiber; 13.5 g protein; 9 g sugar (0 added)

Peanut Noodles with Confetti Veggies and Chicken

NUMBER OF POWER PLANTS: 6

SERVES 3

Just like your favorite Thai takeout joint makes it, but brimming with protein and fiber for a quarter of the price.

INGREDIENTS

6 ounces dry whole-wheat spaghetti or 100% buckwheat soba noodles

¼ cup diced mango or halved grapes

¼ cup no-sugar-added, no-salt-added peanut butter

2 tablespoons + 1 teaspoon naturally brewed tamari (soy sauce) or coconut aminos

2 tablespoons rice vinegar

Juice of 1 lime (2 tablespoons)

1½ teaspoons toasted, unrefined sesame oil

6 ounces finely diced or shredded precooked chicken breast (about 1 breast)

1 cup thinly sliced snow peas (or finely diced English cucumber)

1 cup shredded carrot (or shredded red cabbage)

¼ cup salted dry-roasted peanuts, whole or chopped

3 tablespoons loosely packed fresh cilantro leaves

DIRECTIONS

1. Prepare the noodles (in salted water) per package directions.

2. Meanwhile, in a blender, purée the mango, peanut butter, tamari, vinegar, lime juice, and sesame oil until creamy, about 1 minute. Pour into a large mixing bowl.

3. Drain the noodles, reserving ¼ cup of the pasta liquid. Toss noodles with ice cubes to cool and, when ice cubes are melted, drain the noodles well.

4. Add the noodles to the sauce and toss with tongs to fully coat. If a saucier consistency is desired, add preferred amount of reserved cooking liquid. Add the chicken, snow peas, and carrot to the peanut noodles and toss to combine. Adjust seasoning.

5. Transfer to a serving bowl, and sprinkle with the peanuts and cilantro leaves. If desired, serve with natural sriracha sauce and/or additional tamari on the side.

Make it vegan: Use plant-based chicken instead of the chicken breast.

The numbers: 590 calories; 10 g fiber; 38 g protein; 7 g sugar (0 added)

Tex-Mex Tortilla, Bean, and Sweet Potato Stew

NUMBER OF POWER PLANTS: 9

SERVES 3

Yes, it's called a "stew," but this hearty dish from the border country is light enough to serve in the middle of July.

INGREDIENTS

2 tablespoons avocado oil or sunflower oil

2 sweet potatoes, trimmed, scrubbed, and cut into 1-inch cubes

1 small or ½ large red onion, cut into 1-inch cubes

1 cup frozen corn kernels, thawed and patted dry

1 small jalapeño pepper, with or without seeds, minced

½ teaspoon chili powder

¼ teaspoon + ⅛ teaspoon sea salt, or to taste

¼ teaspoon ground cumin

1 (15-ounce) can no-salt-added black beans, rinsed and drained

1 (14.5-ounce) can diced roasted tomatoes with green chilies (do not drain)

3½ cups low-sodium chicken or vegetable broth

Juice of 1 lime (2 tablespoons) + 3 lime wedges

¼ cup chopped fresh cilantro

2 ounces unsalted yellow corn tortilla chips, coarsely broken, divided

½ cup nonfat plain Greek yogurt*

1 large Hass avocado, pitted, peeled, and diced

DIRECTIONS

1. Heat the oil in a stockpot over medium-high heat. Add the sweet potatoes and onion and sauté until they're lightly browned, about 8 minutes. Add the corn and jalapeño and sauté until the corn begins to brown, about 2½ minutes. Stir in the chili powder, salt, and cumin.

2. Add the beans, tomatoes, broth, and lime juice; bring to a boil over high. Reduce heat to medium and simmer, uncovered, until the sweet potato is fully softened, about 12 minutes. Stir in the cilantro and half of the tortilla chips. Adjust seasoning.

3. Ladle the stew into large bowls, top with yogurt, remaining tortilla chips, and the avocado, and serve with the lime wedges.

*For an extra-thick yogurt topping, strain the yogurt through a cheesecloth- or paper towel–lined mesh strainer at the beginning of stew prep time. Also try a plant-based alternative, such as an almond- or chickpea-based Greek-style yogurt.

The numbers: 660 calories; 18 g fiber; 26 g protein; 13 g sugar (0 added)

Jumbo Turkey Meatballs on Bed of Greens

POWER PLANTS: 9

SERVES 2

You can certainly serve these meatballs over pasta, but they're so rich and filling that they can stand out on their own without the typical carbohydrate coverage.

INGREDIENTS

8 ounces cremini mushrooms

⅔ cup old-fashioned rolled oats

⅓ cup walnut pieces

2 large garlic cloves, peeled and chopped

½ cup packed fresh basil leaves

8 ounces ground turkey (about 93% lean)

¼ cup + 3 tablespoons marinara or arrabbiata sauce, divided

1 tablespoon chia seeds

1 teaspoon fennel seeds

¼ teaspoon + ⅛ teaspoon sea salt, or to taste

½ teaspoon freshly ground black pepper

2 tablespoons extra-virgin olive oil, divided

7 ounces chopped fresh leafy greens, such as kale, spinach, or chard leaves

2 teaspoons balsamic vinegar

2 tablespoons shredded parmesan cheese

DIRECTIONS

1. Preheat the oven to 425°F. Line a rimmed baking sheet with parchment paper or a silicone baking mat.

2. Add the mushrooms, oats, walnuts, garlic, and basil to a food processor and pulse until well crumbled. Transfer to a large mixing bowl. Add the ground turkey, ¼ cup of the marinara sauce, the chia seeds, fennel seeds, salt, and pepper, and stir until evenly combined.

3. Form into 4 jumbo-size meatballs, about ¾ cup mixture each. Arrange on the baking sheet and brush the meatballs with 1 tablespoon of the olive oil. Roast for 15 minutes, flip them over, and roast until well done, about 15 minutes more. Brush (using a clean brush) with the remaining 3 tablespoons marinara sauce and return to the oven to heat through, about 2 minutes more.

4. Meanwhile, heat the remaining 1 tablespoon olive oil in a large, deep skillet over medium heat, and add the leafy greens. Toss until just wilted (timing varies). Stir in the balsamic vinegar. Season with salt, if desired.

5. Arrange the greens on a platter or individual plates, top with the meatballs, and sprinkle with the parmesan cheese. Serve.

The numbers: 670 calories; 10 g fiber; 38 g protein; 6 g sugar (0 added)

Pesto, Sausage, and
Salad Flatbread Pizza

POWER PLANTS: 5

SERVES 2

Faster, cheaper, and more nutritious than the discs from your average delivery joint.

INGREDIENTS

3 tablespoons deli-prepared or jarred basil pesto

2 (2.5-ounce) whole grain naan or pocketless pitas

⅓ cup shredded part-skim mozzarella cheese

3 tablespoons shelled, lightly salted pistachios, chopped, divided

3½ ounces precooked Italian turkey or chicken sausage link(s), no antibiotics, cut into coins

10 cherry or grape tomatoes, various colors, sliced

1½ teaspoons lemon juice

½ teaspoon grated lemon zest, or to taste

2 teaspoons extra-virgin olive oil

1½ cups (1.5 ounces) packed fresh baby arugula leaves

¼ teaspoon freshly ground black pepper

DIRECTIONS

1. Preheat the oven to 450°F. Place a baking sheet in the oven.
2. Evenly spread the pesto onto the two naan or pitas. Top (to the edges) with the mozzarella, half of the pistachios, all the sausage, and tomatoes.
3. Remove the hot baking sheet from oven; carefully transfer the topped naan to the baking sheet; and bake until the cheese is melted, toppings are steamy, and the bottom crust is crisp and browned, about 10 minutes.
4. Meanwhile, whisk together the lemon juice, lemon zest, and olive oil in a medium mixing bowl. Add the arugula and toss to coat.

5. Remove the naan pizzas from the oven and transfer to plates. Pile high with the arugula salad, sprinkle with the remaining pistachios and black pepper, and serve. Enjoy with a fork and knife!

Make it vegan: Use plant-based versions of pesto, sausage, and cheese.

The numbers: 520 calories; 9 g fiber; 25 g protein; 7 g sugar (1 added)

Creole Red Beans Freek-Out

POWER PLANTS: 9

SERVES 3

What is freekeh? It sounds weird and exotic, but it's really not; it's just an ancient grain from Egypt that's grown in popularity in the United States over the past decade or so. You can use another whole grain or riced cauliflower for this recipe, but freekeh just adds one more Power Plant to your growing arsenal.

INGREDIENTS

- 2 teaspoons extra-virgin olive oil
- 2 (3.5-ounce) links uncooked spicy poultry sausage, cut into coins
- 1 medium green bell pepper, seeded and cut into small cubes
- 1 small yellow onion, peeled and diced
- 1 medium celery stalk, finely diced
- 3 large garlic cloves, peeled and finely chopped
- 1 (15-ounce) can kidney beans, drained
- ½ cup low-sodium vegetable or chicken broth
- 1 large fully ripened beefsteak tomato, seeded and diced
- 1½ teaspoons no-salt-added Creole or Cajun seasoning, or to taste
- ¼ teaspoon + ⅛ teaspoon sea salt, or to taste
- 1 teaspoon red wine vinegar
- ¾ teaspoon minced fresh thyme leaves
- 1½ cups cooked freekeh, farro, or sautéed riced cauliflower, warm
- 2 scallions, extra thinly sliced on the diagonal

DIRECTIONS

1. Heat the oil in a large saucepan or deep-sided skillet over medium-high heat. Add the sausage, bell pepper, onion, and celery and cook, stirring occasionally, until the sausage is cooked through and browned and onion is lightly caramel-

ized, about 8 minutes. Add the garlic and sauté until fragrant, about 30 seconds.

2. Stir in the kidney beans, broth, tomato, Creole seasoning, and salt. Cover, reduce heat to medium-low, and simmer until the flavors are blended and mixture is stew-like, about 10 minutes, stirring once halfway through. Stir in the vinegar and thyme. Adjust seasoning.

3. Ladle the stew-like bean mixture alongside the freekeh, top with the scallion, and serve.

Make it vegan: Use plant-based sausage instead of chicken or turkey sausage.

The numbers: 610 calories; 15 g fiber; 30 g protein; 6 g sugar (0 added)

Eggplant Steaks with Velvety Sun-Dried Tomato Sauce

POWER PLANTS: 6

SERVES 2

High-protein tofu, quinoa, and edamame make this vegan dish a rich, hearty meal. You won't miss the meat!

INGREDIENTS

  1 large (about 22 ounces) eggplant, trimmed and cut lengthwise into 6 slices

  2 tablespoons extra-virgin olive oil, divided

  ¼ teaspoon sea salt, or to taste

  2 large garlic cloves, peeled and sliced

  1¼ cups low-sodium vegetable broth, or as desired

  Juice and zest of ½ small lemon (1 tablespoon juice), divided

  1 cup sun-dried tomatoes, chopped

  8 ounces organic silken tofu

  1⅓ cups cooked quinoa, warm

  ¼ cup dry-roasted edamame or 2 tablespoons pan-toasted pine nuts

  ¼ cup packed small or torn fresh basil leaves

DIRECTIONS

1. Preheat oven to 450°F. Line a large baking sheet with parchment paper or a silicone baking mat. Arrange eggplant slices on the baking sheet; brush the top sides only with 1½ tablespoons of the olive oil and sprinkle with salt. Roast until fully cooked through and lightly browned, no flipping or rotating required, about 23 minutes.

2. Meanwhile, heat the remaining ½ tablespoon oil in a medium saucepan over medium heat. Add the garlic and sauté until fragrant, about 1 minute. Add the vegetable broth, lemon juice, and sun-dried tomatoes; increase heat to high; and bring to a boil. Then reduce heat to medium-low and simmer until the tomatoes are fully softened, about 5 minutes.

3. Add the simmered sun-dried tomato mixture and tofu to a blender. Cover and purée until creamy, at least 3 minutes on high speed. Transfer the sauce back to the saucepan, adjust seasoning, and keep warm until ready to serve. If desired, stir in additional broth for a thinner consistency.

4. Spread three-quarters of the sauce onto two rimmed plates, top with the eggplant steaks and quinoa, and dollop with the remaining sauce. Sprinkle with the roasted edamame, lemon zest, and fresh basil; serve.

The numbers: 610 calories; 23 g fiber; 27 g protein; 32 g sugar (0 added)

Sheet Pan-Roasted Veggies and Tempeh with Tahini Sauce

POWER PLANTS: 6

SERVES 2

To save time, consider making the tahini sauce up to a week in advance and keep chilled. It's not a bad idea to be constantly roasting vegetables as well; you can keep a refrigerated arsenal on hand and quickly zap them for side dishes.

INGREDIENTS

- 1 (8-ounce) package tempeh, cut crosswise into ½-inch slices (about 16 slices)
- 1 pound (about 5 cups total) veggie mixture, such as halved brussels sprouts and purple or white cauliflower florets
- 1 tablespoon + 1 teaspoon extra-virgin olive oil
- ½ teaspoon sea salt
- ½ teaspoon ground cinnamon
- ¼ teaspoon freshly ground black pepper
- ¼ teaspoon ground cumin
- 1 cup cooked red or white quinoa or whole grain of choice, warm
- Lemony Tahini Sauce (see page 204)
- 1 tablespoon harissa sauce or 1 small extra thinly sliced red hot chili pepper
- 3 tablespoons crisp roasted chickpeas or sliced almonds, toasted
- ¼ cup loosely packed fresh mint leaves

DIRECTIONS

1. Preheat the oven to 425°F. Line a large rimmed baking sheet with unbleached parchment paper or a silicone baking mat.
2. In a large mixing bowl, add tempeh slices, brussels sprouts, cauliflower, and olive oil, and toss to combine. Sprinkle with

salt, cinnamon, black pepper, and cumin, and toss to combine. Arrange in a single layer on the sheet pan. Roast until veggies and tempeh are browned and cooked through, about 25 minutes. Adjust seasoning.

3. Spread quinoa out as a "bed" on individual plates and pile high with the veggies and tempeh. Drizzle everything with all of the tahini sauce; sprinkle with the harissa, chickpeas, and mint; serve.

The numbers (includes sauce): 660 calories; 13 g fiber; 39 g protein; 7 g sugar (1 added)

LEMONY TAHINI SAUCE

3 tablespoons tahini
Juice of 1 lemon (3 tablespoons juice)
2 to 3 tablespoons unsweetened green tea or water, or to desired consistency
1 garlic clove, peeled and minced
Pinch sea salt

In a jar or a liquid measuring cup, shake or whisk together all ingredients. Make up to 1 week in advance and store in a jar in the fridge.

One-Skillet Coconut Curry Chicken Thighs and Vegetable Trio

POWER PLANTS: 6
SERVES 2
Substitute in your favorite vegetables, or whatever you have taking up space in the fridge. The more variety, the better.

INGREDIENTS

1 tablespoon extra-virgin olive oil, divided

14 ounces (about 4 small or 3 medium) organic boneless, skinless chicken thighs

1¼ teaspoons curry powder

½ teaspoon ginger powder

3 cups (6 ounces) broccoli florets

1 large (10-ounce) yellow summer squash, halved lengthwise, then cut crosswise into ½-inch slices

1 large red or orange bell pepper, seeded and cubed, or ¾ cup sliced rainbow chard stems

½ teaspoon + ⅛ teaspoon sea salt, or to taste

⅔ cup low-sodium chicken or vegetable broth

⅓ cup unsweetened organic light coconut milk

Juice of ½ lime (1 tablespoon juice) + wedges of ½ lime

⅓ cup dry whole wheat couscous

3 tablespoons roasted or unroasted cashews

3 tablespoons fresh cilantro leaves

DIRECTIONS

1. Heat 1 teaspoon of the olive oil in a wok or extra-large, deep nonstick skillet over medium-high heat. Add the chicken thighs, curry powder, and ginger powder and cook until well done, about 4 to 5 minutes per side. Transfer to a rimmed plate.

2. In the wok or skillet, in any remaining fat or browned bits, heat the remaining 2 teaspoons olive oil over medium-high heat. Add the broccoli, summer squash, and bell pepper, and sauté until browned and tender yet firm to the bite, about 5 minutes.

3. Return the chicken (and all residual juices) to the wok or skillet. Season the chicken and vegetables with salt. Add the broth and coconut milk and bring just to a boil, then reduce heat to medium-low and simmer until desired stew-like consistency, about 4 minutes. Stir in the lime juice. Adjust seasoning.

4. Meanwhile, prepare the couscous per package directions.

5. Arrange the cooked couscous, chicken, and vegetables into individual bowls. Top with all the curry broth, sprinkle with the cashews and cilantro, and serve with the lime wedges.

The numbers: 620 calories; 9 g fiber; 47 g protein; 13 g sugar (0 added)

Wild Sesame Tuna Steaks with Scallion and Purple Sweet Potato Sauté

POWER PLANTS: 4

SERVES 2

The purple vegetables give this meal a cool, Instagrammable vibe, but you can use the orange versions if that's all your local store carries.

INGREDIENTS

1½ tablespoons peanut or avocado oil, divided

1 (12-ounce) purple sweet potato, scrubbed, trimmed, and cut into ¾-inch cubes, or 12 ounces purple carrot slices

2 scallions, cut into large 1½-inch pieces on the diagonal

½ teaspoon grated fresh gingerroot

1 small red hot chili pepper, seeded and extra thinly sliced

¼ teaspoon sea salt, or to taste, divided

2 (5-ounce) boneless wild yellowfin or other tuna steaks

1½ teaspoons toasted sesame oil

3 tablespoons mixture of unroasted white and black sesame seeds, or to coat

1 cup (1 ounce) packed fresh wild greens or baby arugula

Sweet Tamari Vinaigrette (see page 207)

DIRECTIONS

1. Heat 1 tablespoon of the peanut oil in a wok or large cast-iron or nonstick skillet over medium-high heat. Add the sweet potato and sauté until cooked through and browned, about

10 minutes. Add the scallions, ginger, chili pepper, and ⅛ teaspoon of salt and sauté until the scallions are lightly browned, 2 minutes more.

2. Meanwhile, brush the tuna steaks with the sesame oil; dip entire surface of each steak into the sesame seeds; and sprinkle with the remaining ⅛ teaspoon salt. Fully heat the remaining ½ tablespoon peanut oil in a large cast-iron skillet over medium-high heat, and sear the tuna to desired doneness, about 1 to 1½ minutes per side or until medium rare.

3. Arrange the greens on a platter or individual plates, and top with the tuna (ideally sliced!) and sweet potato mixture. Drizzle everything with the Sweet Tamari Vinaigrette to serve.

The numbers (including vinaigrette): 550 calories; 8 g fiber; 42 g protein; 14 g sugar (5 added)

SWEET TAMARI VINAIGRETTE

1½ tablespoons rice vinegar

1 tablespoon naturally brewed tamari (soy sauce) or coconut aminos, or to taste

2 teaspoons coconut nectar, date syrup, or honey

In a small jar, shake together all ingredients. Store in the refrigerator until ready to use.

Thai-Style Halibut with Mango Relish and Bok Choy

POWER PLANTS: 6

SERVES 2

Halibut is one of the most sustainable fish in American waters, and it's high in healthy omega-3 fatty acids, so it's a terrific choice for folks who don't like the oily taste of other omega-3–rich fish such as tuna or mackerel.

INGREDIENTS

- 1 tablespoon + 2 teaspoons sunflower or peanut oil, divided
- 2 scallions, thinly sliced, green and white parts divided
- 1 small Thai chili pepper or ½ small jalapeño, seeded and minced
- 1 small or ½ large ripe mango, peeled, pitted, and cut into ½-inch cubes (1 cup)
- 1½ teaspoons naturally brewed tamari (soy sauce) or coconut aminos, divided
- 2 teaspoons lime juice + ½ teaspoon grated lime zest, divided
- 2 heads baby bok choy (about 6.5 ounces each), halved lengthwise, rinsed well, and patted dry
- ¼ teaspoon sea salt, or to taste, divided
- 2 (5.5-ounce) halibut or barramundi fillets, patted dry
- 1½ tablespoons sliced almonds, toasted
- 2 tablespoons fresh cilantro leaves or small basil leaves

DIRECTIONS

1. Heat 2 teaspoons of the oil in a medium nonstick skillet over medium heat. Add the white part of the scallions and sauté until the scallions begin to caramelize, about 3 minutes. Add the chili pepper, mango, and ½ teaspoon of the tamari and cook, while stirring occasionally, until the mango is softened, about

7 minutes. Stir in the lime juice and green parts of the scallions, transfer to a bowl, and set aside.

2. Heat 1 teaspoon of the oil in a large nonstick skillet over medium-high heat. Add the bok choy and sauté until lightly browned, about 2 to 2½ minutes per side. Sprinkle with ⅛ teaspoon of the salt and the remaining 1 teaspoon tamari. Transfer to a platter, loosely cover with foil, and keep in a warm spot.

3. Season the fish with the remaining ⅛ teaspoon salt. Heat the remaining 2 teaspoons oil in a large nonstick skillet over medium-high heat; add the fish; and sear undisturbed until a golden-brown crust forms on the bottom, about 3½ minutes. Flip the fillets over, reduce heat to medium, and sear until the fish is cooked through and easily flakes, about 3 minutes more.

4. On the platter, serve fillets alongside the bok choy. Top the fillets with the mango relish. Sprinkle everything with the lime zest, almonds, and cilantro, and serve.

Note: If preferred, grill instead of sautéing the fish fillets and bok choy. Simply brush with oil before grilling over direct medium-high heat.

The numbers: 520 calories; 5 g fiber; 29 g protein; 14 g sugar (0 added)

Grilled Citrus Pork Loin Chops and Charred Green Vegetables

POWER PLANTS: 7

SERVES 2

Any red meat can become a health food if you move a whole bunch of green vegetables into its neighborhood.

INGREDIENTS

Juice and zest of 1 small orange (⅓ cup juice) + 1 medium orange, sliced

Juice of ½ small lemon (1 tablespoon juice) + ½ small lemon, sliced

2 tablespoons extra-virgin olive oil, divided

1 teaspoon Dijon mustard

½ teaspoon minced fresh rosemary leaves + 2 small rosemary sprigs

½ teaspoon sea salt, or to taste, divided

¼ teaspoon freshly ground black pepper, or to taste

2 (6-ounce) lean pasture-raised/heritage (i.e., without antibiotics) boneless center-cut pork loin chops

12 ounces green vegetables (ideally choose two), such as asparagus spears, long zucchini slices, and/or broccolini

1½ cups cooked whole grains, such as barley, spelt, or black rice, warm, or 2 whole grain rolls

½ teaspoon poppy seeds or 1 tablespoon finely chopped pecans

⅛ teaspoon dried hot pepper flakes (optional)

DIRECTIONS

1. In a medium bowl, whisk together the orange zest, orange juice, lemon juice, 1 tablespoon of the olive oil, the mustard, rosemary leaves, ¼ teaspoon of the salt, and the pepper. Add the pork chops to a sealable glass storage container, slowly

pour the marinade on top, and let marinate in the refrigerator for about 1 hour.

2. Remove the pork from the marinade and discard the marinade (or boil the marinade for a few minutes and use as a drizzle sauce).

3. Prepare and preheat the grill or a grill pan. Brush the green vegetables and orange and lemon slices with the remaining 1 tablespoon olive oil. Grill the vegetables, citrus slices, and pork over direct medium-high heat until rich grill marks form and the pork is medium done, about 8 minutes total for the veggies and citrus and 11 minutes total for the pork (minimum internal temperature of 145°F). Sprinkle the pork and veggies with the remaining ¼ teaspoon salt. Adjust seasoning.

4. On a platter or individual plates, serve the pork chops alongside the charred green vegetables and steamed whole grains. Top everything with the grilled citrus slices, poppy seeds, and, if desired, hot pepper flakes. Garnish with the small rosemary sprigs and serve.

The numbers (includes ½ marinade as topping): 480 calories; 11 g fiber; 47 g protein; 12 g sugar (0 added)

Double Butternut Squash Power Pasta with Kale

POWER PLANTS: 7

SERVES 2

"Pulse" pastas are made from alternative starch sources such as lentils, quinoa, or chickpeas. I personally find the chickpea pastas far superior to those made from other plants.

INGREDIENTS

5 ounces dry chickpea pasta shapes, like penne or rotini

1 tablespoon extra-virgin olive oil

9 ounces fresh butternut squash, peeled and cut into ¾-inch cubes (2 cups cubed)

2 garlic cloves, peeled and minced

4 ounces fresh kale, chopped

1½ teaspoons nutritional yeast flakes

1½ teaspoons white wine vinegar

¾ teaspoon sea salt, or to taste

⅛ teaspoon dried hot pepper flakes, or to taste

1 (15-ounce) can unsalted butternut squash purée

1½ ounces plant-based goat cheese or soft vegan tree nut cheese of choice

2 tablespoons raw pepitas or pine nuts

¼ cup loosely packed fresh basil leaves

DIRECTIONS

1. Cook the pasta (in salted water) according to package directions.

2. Meanwhile, in an extra-large, deep nonstick skillet or wok, heat the olive oil over medium-high heat. Add the butternut squash cubes and toss with tongs occasionally until browned and firm yet just cooked through, about 8 minutes. Add the garlic and cook, stirring until fragrant, about 30 seconds. Add the kale, nutritional yeast, vinegar, salt, and hot pepper flakes and toss with tongs until the kale is wilted, about 2 minutes.

3. Drain the pasta well, reserving 1 cup of the pasta water. Add the pasta water and the squash purée into the kale mixture and stir until combined and heated through, about 2 minutes. Add the pasta and stir until desired sauce consistency, about 1 to 2 minutes. Adjust seasoning.

4. Transfer the pasta mixture to pasta bowls; sprinkle with the plant-based cheese, pepitas, and basil; serve.

The numbers: 590 calories; 17 g fiber; 26 g protein; 8 g sugar (0 added)

Berry Good Ricotta

NUMBER OF POWER PLANTS: 5

SERVES 8

What if you could make a dessert from scratch that had all the muscle-nourishing whey protein power of a bodybuilding supplement, plus all the various plant fibers that your microbiome craved—and on the very first bite, you'd immediately start thinking about seconds? This is that impossible dessert. Yes, it's high in sugar—a bit more than you'll get from a scoop of vanilla ice cream. The difference is that much of the sugar comes from fruit.

I fully recommend you use store-bought ricotta for this dish, because you have a life to live. But I also recognize that some of us are adventurous, so I've included a recipe for homemade ricotta.

INGREDIENTS (HOMEMADE RICOTTA)

> **2 quarts whole milk**
> **1 quart heavy cream**
> **1 tablespoon salt**
> **½ cup lemon juice**
> **½ cup white wine vinegar**
> **½ cup buttermilk**

INGREDIENTS (TOPPINGS)

> **1 cup chopped strawberries**
> **1 cup blueberries**
> **¼ cup water**
> **12 mint leaves**
> **3 peaches, halved, pitted, and sliced**
> **24 cherries, halved and pitted**

DIRECTIONS (HOMEMADE RICOTTA)

1. Pour milk, cream, and salt into a large pot, leaving room at the top.

2. Heat over medium heat while stirring constantly to avoid scorching. The temperature should reach a point at which the liquids are simmering but not boiling (about 180°F).
3. Add lemon juice, vinegar, and buttermilk.
4. Turn off the heat, stir once to disperse the acids, and then leave it to separate and cool.
5. Strain through a sieve or colander lined with cheesecloth.

DIRECTIONS (TOPPINGS)

1. Place strawberries, blueberries and water into a blender and blend until smooth.
2. Stack the mint leaves atop one another, then roll as though you're a Cuban cigar maker. Once you've created the mint cigar, slice the cigar thinly (this is called a chiffonade).
3. Smear 1 cup ricotta onto a plate in a circle, top with 1 tablespoon of the berry blend, pile sliced peaches and cherries into the middle of the plate, and garnish with the mint chiffonade.

The numbers: 472 calories; 5 g fiber; 30 g protein; 11 g sugar (0 added)

12

14 Days of Eating the Full-Body Fat Fix

What will you eat when your 7-Day Challenge is done? A quick look at how simple, delicious, and forgiving this plan can be, and a preview of the foods you'll be enjoying in the days, weeks, and months to come.

Congratulations on making it through the gauntlet of the 7-Day Challenge—a week having a whey protein smoothie for breakfast every day, swearing off sweets and refined carbs, limiting whole grains to just one serving per day, and looking high and low for new ways to incorporate thirty Power Plants into your diet.

Of course, as we saw in Chapter 3, it turns out to be a lot easier than it sounds. And, once you learn how to maximize the array of plants in your diet, you open up a whole new world of tastes and flavors, not just for you, but for the 100 trillion microbes living inside you.

But now that the Challenge is over, how should you eat for the rest of your life? Well, all you need to do is to look at every meal with the same three questions in mind:

Where are my Power Plants? (Aim for two or more each meal.)

Where are my Power Proteins? (Look for 25 to 30 grams per meal, and avoid cured meats most of the time.)

Where are my Power Fats? (Dairy, fish, nuts, nut butters, avocado, or olives are top choices.)

If you can't answer those questions, you probably need to add something to your meal to make it complete. A side of guac to go with those tacos, some peppers and onions on top of that pizza, a little container of coleslaw alongside your burger. Making these simple additions, and choosing high-protein, nutritionally diverse meals whenever possible, will help you quell the fire within and set you on the path to a leaner and healthier future.

To get you started, I've outlined a two-week starter plan of perfect eating. Each of these meals has at least 25 grams of protein, healthy fats, and at least two Power Plants. But as we've seen, there are endless variations available, whether you're a pasta lover, a burger meister, or a sushi connoisseur. Try each and every one of these suggested meals, or none of them. But keep those three questions in mind, focus on plant variety, and your microbiome will thank you. (So will the sales team at your favorite store who are going to make nice commissions selling you smaller clothes.)

And remember: Protein for breakfast. Always.

MONDAY

Breakfast:

Jolted Awake whey protein smoothie (recipe, page 57): iced coffee, pine nuts, whole wheat cereal, hemp seeds, frozen banana, peanut butter, cacao powder, and chocolate whey protein.

Lunch:

Turkey and cheddar on whole grain bread with romaine lettuce, mayo, and mustard; side Caesar salad of romaine, pine nuts, and Caesar dressing.

Dinner:

Applebee's Blackened Cajun Salmon with Garlicky Green Beans, Fire-Grilled Veggies, and Fat-Free Dressing.

Dessert:

Small ice cream cone.

TUESDAY

Breakfast:

Two eggs, cheddar, and ham on a Skinny Wheat Bagel from Au Bon Pain.

Lunch:

Popeyes Blackened Tenders (5) with Red Beans & Rice (regular).

Snack:

Apple and cheddar cheese slices.

Dinner:

How Do I Get Rid of All These Tomatoes? (recipe, page 64): salad with fresh heirloom tomatoes, English cucumber, honeydew, pomegranate, basil leaves, and crushed toasted walnuts, served with grilled salmon.

WEDNESDAY

Breakfast:

Whole grain waffle topped with cottage cheese, raspberries, hemp seeds, and pistachios.

Lunch:

Chicken, pepper, onion, and cheese quesadilla with guacamole.

Dinner:

Sheet Pan-Roasted Veggies and Tempeh with Tahini Sauce (recipe, page 203): tempeh, mixed vegetables, quinoa, mint, and roasted chickpeas.

THURSDAY

Breakfast:

Yogurt parfait with 1 cup plain whole-fat Greek yogurt, 1¼ cups frozen mixed berries, ¼ cup walnuts, and 2 tablespoons muesli cereal.

Lunch:

Taco Bell Power Menu Bowl with chicken.

Dinner:

Mixed sushi rolls with a side of edamame or seaweed salad.

Dessert:

Scoop of ricotta cheese with cacao powder and raspberries.

FRIDAY

Breakfast:

My Cherry Amour whey protein smoothie (recipe, page 59): frozen cherries, strawberries, cranberries, cashews, baby spinach, avocado, and chocolate whey protein.

Lunch:

Chipotle Steak Salad with brown rice, black beans, Monterey Jack, salsa, and chipotle honey dressing.

Dinner:

Grilled fish, quinoa, and arugula salad with blueberries, golden berries, and balsamic dressing.

Dessert:

Small bowl of frozen yogurt topped with chopped nuts and berries.

SATURDAY

Breakfast:

Two large eggs, scrambled with mozzarella cheese, roasted potatoes, green pepper, onion, in olive oil, with mixed fruit on the side.

Lunch:

Panera Bread Turkey on Rustic Sourdough and a cup of Ten Vegetable Soup.

Dinner:

One-Skillet Coconut Curry Chicken Thighs and Vegetable Trio (recipe, page 204): chicken thighs with broccoli, summer squash, bell pepper, whole wheat couscous, cashews, and cilantro.

SUNDAY

Breakfast:

High-protein cereal such as Kay's Naturals, Kashi Go Rise, or Special K Protein, with mixed, unsalted nuts, hemp seeds, and 2% milk.

Lunch:

Chick-fil-A Spicy Southwest Salad.

Snack:

Trail mix of nuts and dried apricots.

Dinner:

Tom's Big Game Day Chili (recipe, page 183): beef, turkey, or game meat, whole peeled tomatoes, peppers, onion, kidney and black beans, and brown rice (optional).

MONDAY

Breakfast:

Starbucks Spinach, Feta & Egg White Breakfast Wrap with Rolled & Steel-Cut Oatmeal with Blueberries

Lunch:

Quinoa salad with feta, chickpeas, and mixed vegetables.

Snack:

Almonds and olives.

Dinner:

Whole wheat penne pasta topped with grilled shrimp and vegetables, extra-virgin olive oil, and black pepper.

TUESDAY

Breakfast:

1 cup plain, whole-fat (or 2%) Greek yogurt topped with mixed nuts, chia seeds, and fresh or frozen berries.

Lunch:

Wendy's large chili and a half order Avocado Chicken Salad with Southwest Ranch Dressing.

Dinner:

Cracker Barrel Old Country Store Lemon-Grilled Rainbow Trout with Turnip Greens Bowl.

WEDNESDAY

Breakfast:

1 cup cottage cheese with mixed berries or melon chunks.

Lunch:

Gyro with roasted lamb, grilled vegetables, tahini, and a side of hummus.

Dinner:

The Roast of Brussels salad (recipe, page 66): brussels sprouts, radicchio, Granny Smith apple, dried cherries, scallions, and peanuts, served with grilled pork.

THURSDAY

Breakfast:

Kale to the Chief whey protein smoothie (recipe, page 58): oat or soy milk, kale, parsley, oats, flaxseeds, date, chia seeds, and vanilla whey protein.

Lunch:

Bowl of chicken noodle soup with carrots and celery, plus an apple.

Dinner:

Delivery pizza topped with at least two vegetables, plus a small side chicken Caesar salad.

FRIDAY

Breakfast:

Denny's Loaded Veggie Omelette with seasonal fruit and English muffin.

Lunch:

Subway Turkey Cali Club on whole wheat bread with sliced avocado.

Dinner:

Grilled steaks with a side of frozen sweet potato fries (baked) and coleslaw.

Dessert:

Small ice cream cone.

SATURDAY

Breakfast:

Daiquiris for Breakfast whey protein smoothie (recipe, page 57): Greek yogurt, banana, coconut, peach, pineapple, mandarin orange, mango, raspberries, and vanilla whey protein.

Lunch:

Bowl of multi-bean soup, such as Bob's Red Mill 13-Bean or DeLallo Bean Medley, with grilled cheese sandwich on whole grain toast.

Dinner:

Wild Sesame Tuna Steaks with Scallion and Purple Sweet Potato Sauté (recipe, page 206): tuna with purple sweet potato, ginger, sesame seeds, arugula, and Sweet Tamari Vinaigrette.

Dessert:

Cacao (70% or more) chocolate bar.

SUNDAY

Breakfast:

Whole grain toast with mashed avocado and spices, plus 1 cup Greek yogurt and mixed fruit.

Lunch:

Boston Market turkey breast, bacon brussels sprouts, and corn-bread.

Snack:

Apple slices with peanut butter.

Dinner:

The Butternut Beet salad (recipe, page 65): diced beets, butternut squash, kale, shallot, pepitas, and chives, served with grilled skirt steak.

13

Troubleshooting the Full-Body Fat Fix

Frequently asked questions, simple cheats, and time-saving strategies.

I f inflammation is such a huge problem, why don't we all just take anti-inflammatories every day?

Because while too much inflammation is bad for you, too little is bad for you as well. Inflammation plays an important role in fighting infection, healing wounds, and managing several other major health threats. Dramatically dampening the inflammatory response could set us up for unforeseen and dangerous scenarios, said Shilpa Ravella, MD, gastroenterologist and author of *A Silent Fire*.

"When we take an immune-suppressing drug, there is always a side effect," she told me. "When we block one pathway, another takes over." So for example, while studies of the anti-inflammatory canakinumab show a beneficial impact on heart disease patients, regularly prescribing such drugs could have additional impacts we don't know about yet, such as raising cancer risk. And overuse of over-the-counter oral anti-inflammatories such as aspirin and ibuprofen can have negative effects on the digestive system.

I love that this program is packed with lots of food. But won't eating so much cause me to gain weight?

We've been hoodwinked into thinking that eating more food means gaining more weight. It doesn't. The primary driver of weight gain is inflammation, and the primary driver of inflammation is a lack of nutrients feeding our microbiomes and too many additives causing damage to them. Here's a saying worth keeping in mind: If it's an edible plant, put it in your mouth.

That said, calories—in particular carbohydrate calories—are a contributing factor to weight gain, for sure. If you are not seeing changes as rapidly as you'd like, start by reducing your serving sizes of starchy foods such as grains and root vegetables. If, for example, you might normally eat a full cup of cooked rice, you might want to dial down to ⅔ of a cup. That one tweak will cut 60 to 100 calories, which over time should be enough to spark enhanced weight loss.

I sometimes find myself eating even when I didn't intend to be. Like, *Who put this food in my mouth?* How can I stop instinctively picking up what's lying around, especially at my office?

"Mindless eating" happens all the time: It's what we do when we're at the movies and our hand hits the bottom of the popcorn bucket before we're even through the trailers. That's fine a few times a month while watching Tom Cruise continue to defy gravity, but it's a curse when it happens to us day in and day out.

We eat for a lot of reasons—including managing stress or bonding with others—that have nothing to do with either hunger or nutritional needs. But when you're watching your weight and your health, it helps to watch your hunger levels as well.

One way to shortcut that instinct is to do a quick self-check whenever you find yourself reaching for a bit of food. Rate your level of hunger on a scale of 1 to 10, with 1 being "Trapped in a cave without food for three days" and 10 being that exploding gluttonous man from *Monty Python's The Meaning of Life*. If you feel hungry—maybe in the 4 or 5 range, then grab a bite; don't wait to eat until you hit a 1 or a 2. And if you're more in the 6 or 7 range, feeling not stuffed but satisfied, then it's time to stop eating.

Getting enough protein at breakfast is hard, and I don't necessarily want to have to make a protein smoothie every morning. What else can I eat to get my 25 to 30 grams of protein in the morning?

Here are some other ways to hit that number:

1 cup cottage cheese (25 g)

2 packets instant oatmeal (8 g) in 1 cup milk (8 g) with 1 ounce chopped almonds (5 g) and 2 tablespoons hemp seeds (7 g)

½ whole wheat bagel (5 g) with 2 tablespoons cream cheese (2 g) and 3 ounces lox (15 g), plus 1 ounce pumpkin seeds (5 g)

1 cup plain Greek yogurt (20 g) with 2 tablespoons ground flaxseeds (3 g), berries, and ¼ cup unsalted mixed nuts (6 g)

Breakfast burrito with ¾ cup chopped, scrambled tofu (15 g) with 1 ounce cheese (5 g) and ½ cup pinto beans (4.5 g) in a whole grain flour tortilla (1 g)

2 tablespoons peanut butter (7 g) and a sliced banana (1.5 g) on two slices of whole wheat toast (8 g), washed down with 1 cup milk (8 g)

Is there a way to increase my protein intake while still focusing on eating a "plant-based" diet?

Remember that "plant-based" doesn't mean "plant-only." In many cases, it means just eating fewer meats and other animal products and substituting in more plant foods. But even if you were to go vegetarian, there are plenty of ways to ensure you're getting enough protein.

When eating plants only, it's important to combine foods to get a complete set of amino acids—the building blocks of muscle and other tissue. Animal-based foods, including eggs, meat, fish, and dairy, already come with the complete set of aminos (there are sixteen in all). Some plants also offer a complete set: quinoa; soy (including tempeh, tofu, and edamame); seitan (similar to tempeh, it's made from wheat gluten); buckwheat; pumpkin seeds; hemp seeds; and sprouted grain bread are all complete proteins.

Otherwise, a solid rule of thumb is to combine whole grains (brown rice, oats, whole wheat, corn) with legumes, nuts, and seeds (beans, lentils, peanut butter, chia seeds, sunflower seeds). In many cases, traditional ethnic vegetarian foods evolved with us for just this reason: A whole wheat pasta with a pesto made from pine nuts is a whole protein. So is hummus and pita; beans and rice; even peanut butter and jelly on whole grain bread.

You can also opt for plant-based protein powders. Just make sure to choose a "complete" protein—one made from a variety of plant proteins—rather than one derived from a single plant. In addition, check the label to make sure it includes leucine, an amino acid that helps stimulate muscle growth but one that's often missing from plant-based protein powders.

Is there a simple way to tell whether a packaged food is good for me or bad for me?

More and more evidence tells us that the emulsifiers, preservatives, artificial sweeteners, and other nonfood substances in packaged foods can damage the microbiome. It doesn't matter if the label on the front says "natural," "keto," or "artisanal." Those are just marketing terms. In one small study, subjects were put on a diet of either whole foods (lean meats, produce, whole grains) or ultra-processed foods (packaged snacks, baked goods, cured meats). The participants were presented with the same amount of total calories, protein, and carbs, and allowed to consume as much as they wanted. Then, after two weeks, the two groups of volunteers switched off, with the whole foods group eating ultra-processed foods, and vice versa. The researchers discovered that on the ultra-processed diet, subjects ate an average of 500 calories more per day than they did when on the whole-foods diet. They also gained an average of two pounds during their two weeks of eating packaged foods, and they lost an average of two pounds during their time eating whole foods.

That said, unless you have a kitchen staff the size of a football team, there are plenty of foods that you're going to want to buy premade. To find the absolute healthiest products, turn over the package and look at the nutrition label on the back. Then use this simple math equation:

Protein + Fiber > Sugar

So, if the total number of protein grams plus the total number of fiber grams is greater than the total number of sugar grams, you've probably got a relatively healthy food. If that's not the case, put it back and keep shopping.

For example, take Chobani Low-Fat Plain Greek Yogurt. At 130 calories, 0 g fiber, 17 g protein, and just 4 g sugar in a ¾-cup serving, it's a great choice.

But what happens when Chobani tries to fancy its product up with something that sounds healthy? Chobani 2% Mango on the Bottom Greek Yogurt also has 130 calories per serving. But it has 0 fiber, 11 g protein, and a whopping 14 grams of sugar. So, while the plain yogurt has more protein than sugar, the flavored product flips that script.

This works for just about every product on the shelves. For example:

Thomas' Cinnamon Raisin English Muffin
4 g protein + 2 g fiber = 6 g
8 g sugar

Yikes! This breakfast food has more sugar than protein and fiber combined! But just look a little deeper in the bread aisle:

Thomas' Whole Wheat English Muffin
5 g protein + 3 g fiber = 8 g
1 g sugar

See how clear the difference is? Do this easy math on every packaged food you pick up, and you'll soon turn your shopping cart into a steamroller of nutritional power.

I understand why I should cut out sweetened drinks and artificially sweetened drinks. But I don't love the taste of plain water. What else can I drink?

Unsweetened teas are a great choice, and many companies make high-end seltzers that are packed with flavor yet with zero calories. Or, consider pouring a shot of 100 percent real fruit juice (cranberry, pomegranate, or blackberry, for example) over ice in a tall glass, and filling the rest of the glass with plain sparkling water. You'll be hooked!

I'm not big on cooking, but I want to eat more fresh foods. Any tips on kitchen prep?

Cooking up foods in advance is a great way to ensure that you're stocked with the healthiest options. In just a couple of hours on a weekend afternoon you could whip up just about everything you need for the next seven days. Start by cooking up some whole grains: Brown rice, quinoa, or other grains can be cooked and refrigerated to serve as a ground floor for upcoming meals. You can do the same with beans if you prefer making them from scratch. You can also throw a whole bunch of proteins on the grill on a sunny day, then refrigerate and use as the anchors to a meal or sliced on top of salads.

For vegetables like broccoli, cauliflower, and asparagus, start by flashing them in a pot of boiling water to bring out their colors and flavors: First, cut the vegetables into large chunks. Boil the water with a touch of salt, then throw in a handful of the cut vegetables. Wait a moment or two until the water returns to a boil, then scoop them out and immediately immerse them in a pot of ice water to stop the cooking process. You'll see that the vegetables have brightened up a bit. Now drain the vegetables thoroughly (I like to flash boil vegetables in the morning and then let them dry in a strainer for several hours). You can then spread them on a roasting pan, drizzle with olive oil and salt, and roast them in the oven at 400°F for about 30 minutes, or until soft.

I know there's no such thing as a "superfood," but are there any foods we commonly overlook and should eat more of?

Some of the most insanely nutritious foods are also some of our least celebrated:

Black pepper: Whenever your waiter says, "Would you like pepper on that?" your answer should be yes. A 2022 study found that piperine, the active compound in black pepper, "provides therapeutic benefits in patients suffering from diabetes, obesity, arthritis, oral cancer, breast cancer, multiple myeloma, metabolic syndrome, hypertension, Parkinson's disease, Alzheimer's disease, cerebral stroke, cardiovascular diseases, kidney diseases, inflammatory diseases, and rhinopharyngitis." How's that for grinding down your health risks?

Watercress: It may sound fancy, but watercress is one of the least expensive salad ingredients you can find in the market. (It's sometimes sold alongside lettuces; other stores sell it alongside the fresh herbs.) A cruciferous vegetable, it packs all the benefits of other similar foods like kale or broccoli, but with an extra punch: Watercress helps to reverse DNA damage and may be a secret weapon for former smokers concerned about lowering their cancer risk, according to a study in the *American Journal of Clinical Nutrition*.

Parsley: You know that leafy thing you leave on the side of your plate at the end of your meal? Eat it. Parsley is not only a natural breath-freshener, but animal studies indicate it may have "a remarkable antidepressant-like" effect, wrote the authors of a study in the journal *Molecules*.

Grocery prices are insane. How can I eat healthy while saving money?

When you walk into any supermarket anywhere in America, the first thing you'll see is the fresh produce aisle. Do you think corporations put it right up front because the profit margins are low? No. But you can save money and even boost your nutrition factor a bit by heading to the freezer section. Most frozen produce hits the deep freeze within hours of harvest, while what's in the fresh produce section may well have been picked while still unripe and shipped from Mexico, shedding a trail of nutrients all along the way. A study in the *Journal of Agricultural and Food Chemistry* found that the nutrient status of frozen peas, broccoli, carrots, strawberries, spinach, corn, blueberries, and green beans was equal to or greater than that of supposedly fresh supermarket produce, while frozen spinach was nutritionally superior to its fresh counterpart. Plus, frozen produce usually comes in at about half the price of fresh, and it's often easy to find terrific mixes of, say, four different berries or stir-fry vegetables in one bag.

Any tips on buying the freshest produce?

In general, the best fruits and vegetables are often irregularly shaped and blemished. Anything that looks perfect—especially if it's swollen up like a ballplayer on steroids—has probably been heavily treated with pesticides. When you pick up almost any fruit or vegetable, it should feel heavy and sturdy, with a taut skin. Here are some specifics to look for:

Artichokes

Seek out deep-green, heavy artichokes with tightly closed leaves that squeak when pinched together.
Peak: March to May
Storage: In the fridge, in a plastic bag, for up to five days

Asparagus

Look for tight, purple-tinged buds. The thinner the spears, the sweeter and more tender they will be.
Peak: February to June
Storage: Trim the woody ends. Stand the spears in a bit of water in a tall container; cover the tops with a plastic bag. Cook within a few days.

Avocados

Find firm fruit with no sunken, mushy spots and with a waxy, rather than shiny, appearance. Shake it—a rattle means the pit has pulled away from the flesh.
Peak: Year-round
Storage: To ripen, place in a paper bag and store at room temperature for two to four days. Add an apple to the bag to speed up the ripening process. Once the avocado feels ready to eat, you can store it in the fridge for up to one week.

Bell peppers

These should have plenty of heft for their size, and wrinkle-free skin. Stems should be lively green. Note: Red peppers are just green peppers left to ripen on the vine, which means they are richer in nutrients.

Peak: Year-round

Storage: Refrigerate in the crisper for up to two weeks.

Blueberries

You want plump, uniform, indigo berries with taut skin and a dull white frost.

Peak: May to October

Storage: Transfer them unwashed to an airtight container and refrigerate for five to seven days. Wash before eating.

Broccoli

Find rigid stems with tight floret clusters that are deep green or tinged purple. Pass on any with yellowing heads, which signifies that they are turning bitter.

Peak: October to April

Storage: Refrigerate in a plastic bag for up to one week.

Button mushrooms

Find tightly closed, firm caps that aren't slimy or riddled with soft, dark spots.

Peak: September to March

Storage: Spread mushrooms on a flat surface, cover with a damp paper towel, and refrigerate up to three to five days. If the caps are open, with visible gills, eat them sooner.

Eggplant

It should feel heavy and have tight, shiny skin. When pressed, it should feel springy, not spongy. Stem should be bright green.

Peak: August to September

Storage: Keep in a cool location (not the fridge) for up to three days. Eggplants are sensitive to the cold and don't keep well.

Grapes

Find plump, wrinkle-free grapes that are firmly attached to the stems. A silvery white powder ("bloom") means they'll stay fresher longer. Green grapes with a yellowish hue are the sweetest.

Peak: May to October

Storage: Keep unwashed in a shallow bowl in the fridge for up to one week.

Green beans

Good beans have vibrant, smooth surfaces. The best are thin, young, and velvety, and snap when gently bent.

Peak: May to October

Storage: Refrigerate unwashed in an unsealed bag for up to one week.

Kiwis

A ripe kiwi will be slightly yielding to the touch. Avoid mushy or wrinkled ones with an off smell.

Peak: Year-round

Storage: Leave at room temperature to ripen. To quicken the process, place kiwis in a paper bag with an apple or ripe banana. Once ripe, refrigerate in a plastic bag for up to a week.

Papayas

Look for papayas that are starting to turn yellow and yield a bit when lightly squeezed.

Peak: June to September

Storage: Once ripe, eat immediately or refrigerate up to three days. Green papayas should be ripened at room temperature in a dark setting until yellow blotches appear.

Peaches

Good peaches have a fruity aroma and a yellow or warm cream background color, without green shoulders. They're ready when they yield to gentle pressure on the seams.

Peak: May to October

Storage: Leave unripe ones out at room temperature. Ripe ones go in the fridge, but eat them within two to four days.

Pears

You want pleasant fragrances and some softness at the stem end. Some brown discoloration is fine.

Peak: August to March

Storage: Ripen at room temperature in a loosely closed paper bag.

Pineapples

Look for vibrant green leaves, a bit of softness to the fruit, and a sweet fragrance at the stem end. Avoid spongy fruit. A pineapple is ready to be eaten when you can gently tug at a leaf and have it break free.

Peak: March to July

Storage: If it's unripe, keep it at room temperature for three to four days until it softens and gives off a pineapple aroma. Refrigerate for up to five days.

Raspberries

Plump dry berries are best. Look for good shape and intense, uniform color. Flip the box over and look for any leaking at the bottom, which indicates the berries are overripe.

Peak: May to September

Storage: Raspberries get mushy after washing, so store them unwashed in a single layer on a paper towel. Cover with a damp paper towel and refrigerate for two to three days. Wash right before eating.

Romaine lettuce

Look for crisp leaves that are free of browning edges and rust spots.

Peak: Year-round

Storage: Refrigerate for five to seven days in a plastic bag.

Strawberries

Seek out unblemished berries with bright red color that extends right to the stem, and a strong, fruity smell. The feel should be neither hard nor mushy.

Peak: April to September

Storage: Place unwashed berries in a single layer on a paper towel in a covered container and refrigerate.

Tomatoes

Go for heavy ones rich in color and free of wrinkles, bruises, cracks, or soft spots. Note that the majority of a tomato's nutrients are found in the skin, so smaller tomato varieties like grape tomatoes are more potent.

Peak: June to September

Storage: Never in the fridge! Cold destroys a tomato's flavor and texture. Keep on the kitchen counter out of direct sunlight for up to one week.

Watermelon

You want a heavy, dense melon that's free of cuts and sunken areas. The rind should be dull, with a creamy-yellow underside. A slap will produce a hollow thump.

Peak: June to August

Storage: Keep whole in the fridge for up to one week to prevent flesh from drying out and turning fibrous.

Acknowledgments

This book would not have been possible without the ongoing support of dozens of friends, family, and colleagues. Particular thanks to the team at St. Martin's Press, including—but hardly limited to—Elizabeth Beier, Brigitte Dale, Ginny Perrin, John Karle, Brant Janeway, Amelia Beckerman, Lizz Blaise, Michael Storrings, Meryl Levavi, and Elizabeth Degenhard. Thanks to Richard Pine and the team at InkWell Management, and to my colleagues at AARP, especially Myrna Blyth, Bob Love, Neil Wertheimer, and Jodi Lipson. Thanks also to my parents, Lynn Elena Lorenzo-Luaces Perrine and Thomas Charles Deerslayer Perrine. Special thanks to Jackie Newgent, RDN, and Chef Noah Perrine for their extraordinary recipes and culinary advice. And thanks to Bob and Kate Blumer, Jorge Cruise, and Jon Fine and Laurel Touby for their big-brainstorm energy.

And thanks to you, for taking this journey with me.

Studies, Resources, and Further Reading

INTRODUCTION: You're Not Fat, You're on Fire!

Scheithauer, T., Rampanelli, E., et al. "Gut Microbiota as a Trigger for Metabolic Inflammation in Obesity and Type 2 Diabetes." *Frontiers in Immunology (Mucosal Immunity)* 11, no. 571731 (2020). https://doi.org/10.3389/fimmu.2020.571731.

Melamed, Y., Kislev, M., et al. "The Plant Component of an Acheulian Diet at Gesher Benot Ya'aqov, Israel." *PNAS* 113, no. 51 (2016): 14674–14679. https://doi.org/10.1073/pnas.1607872113.

McDonald, D., Hyde, E., et al. "American Gut: An Open Platform for Citizen Science Microbiome Research." *ASM Journals* 3, no. 3 (2018). https://doi.org/10.1128/msystems.00031-18.

Corbin, K., et al. "Host-Diet-Gut Microbiome Interactions Influence Human Energy Balance: a Randomized Clinical Trial." *Nature Communications* 14 (2023): 3161. https://doi.org/10.1038/s41467-023-38778-x.

Spector, T. "Your Gut Bacteria Don't Like Junk Food—Even If You Do." *The Conversation,* May 10, 2015.

Johansen, J., Atarashi, K., Arai, Y., et al. "Centenarians Have a Diverse Gut Virome with the Potential to Modulate Metabolism and Promote Healthy Lifespan." *Nature Microbiology* 8 (2023): 1064–1078. https://doi.org/10.1038/s41564-023-01370-6.

1. How Inflammation Makes Us Sick, Bloated, and Unhappy

Wensveen, F., Valentić, S., et al. "The 'Big Bang' in Obese Fat: Events Initiating Obesity-Induced Adipose Tissue Inflammation." *European Journal of Immunology* 29 (2015): 2446-2456. https://doi.org/10.1002/eji.201545502.

University of Western Ontario. "Your Belly Fat Could Be Making You Hungrier." *Science-Daily*, April 17, 2008. www.sciencedaily.com/releases/2008/04/080416153551.htm. Accessed June 3, 2023.

Yu, J., Choi, W., et al. "Relationship Between Inflammatory Markers and Visceral Obesity in Obese and Overweight Korean Adults." *Medicine (Baltimore)* 98, no. 9 (2019): e14740. https://doi.org/10.1097/MD.0000000000014740.

Baothman, O. A., Zamzami, M. A., Taher, I., et al. "The Role of Gut Microbiota in the Development of Obesity and Diabetes." *Lipids in Health and Disease* 15, no. 108 (2016). https://doi.org/10.1186/s12944-016-0278-4.

Le Roy, C., Kurilshikov, A., et al. "Yoghurt Consumption Is Associated with Changes in the Composition of the Human Gut Microbiome and Metabolome." *BMC Microbiology* 22, no. 39 (2022). https://doi.org/10.1186/s12866-021-02364-2.

Wastyk, H., and Fragiadakis, G. "Gut-Microbiota-Targeted Diets Modulate Human Immune Status." *Cell* 184, no.16 (2021): 4137–4153. http://doi.org/10.1016/j.cell.2021.06.019.

Bentley, R. A., Ormerod, P., and Ruck, D. J. "Recent Origin and Evolution of Obesity-Income Correlation Across the United States." *Palgrave Communications* 4, no. 146 (2018). https://doi.org/10.1057/s41599-018-0201-x.

Santora, M. "Teenagers' Suit Says McDonald's Made Them Obese." *The New York Times*, November 21, 2002: B1.

Urban, L., Weber, J., et al. "Energy Contents of Frequently Ordered Restaurant Meals and Comparison with Human Energy Requirements and US Department of Agriculture Database Information: A Multisite Randomized Study." *Journal of the Academy of Nutrition and Dietetics* 116, no. 4 (2016): 590–598.E6. https://doi.org/10.1016/j.jand.2015.11.009.

French, S. A., Wall, M., and Mitchell, N. R. "Household Income Differences in Food Sources and Food Items Purchased." *International Journal of Behavioral Nutrition and Physical Activity* 7, no. 77 (2010). https://doi.org/10.1186/1479-5868-7-77.

Roberts, S., Das, S., et al. "Measured Energy Content of Frequently Purchased Restaurant Meals: Multi-Country Cross Sectional Study." *BMJ* 363 (2018): k4864. https://doi.org/10.1136/bmj.k4864.

Maurel, M., Castagné, R., et al. "Patterning of Educational Attainment Across Inflammatory Markers: Findings from a Multi-Cohort Study." *Brain, Behavior and Immunology* 90 (2020): 303–310. https://doi.org/10.1016/j.bbi.2020.09.002.

Iyer, H. S., Hart, J. E., James, P., et al. "Impact of Neighborhood Socioeconomic Status, Income Segregation, and Greenness on Blood Biomarkers of Inflammation." *Environment International* 162 (2022): 107164. https://doi.org/10.1016/j.envint.2022.107164.

Xu, F., Earp, J. E., Blissmer, B. J., Lofgren, I. E., Delmonico, M. J., and Greene, G. W. "The Demographic Specific Abdominal Fat Composition and Distribution Trends in US Adults from 2011 to 2018." *International Journal of Environmental Research and Public Health* 19, no. 19 (2022): 12103. https://doi.org/10.3390/ijerph191912103.

2. The Full-Body Fat Fix in Three Simple Steps

Martínez Steele, E., Baraldi, L. G., Louzada, M., et al. "Ultra-Processed Foods and Added Sugars in the US Diet: Evidence from a Nationally Representative Cross-Sectional Study." *BMJ Open* 6, no. 3 (2016): e009892. https://doi.org/10.1136/bmjopen-2015-009892.

Marino, M., Puppo, F., Del Bo', C., Vinelli, V., Riso, P., Porrini, M., and Martini, D. "A Systematic Review of Worldwide Consumption of Ultra-Processed Foods: Findings and Criticisms." *Nutrients* 13, no. 8 (2021): 2778. https://doi.org/10.3390/nu13082778.

"Prevalence of Obesity Among Adults, BMI >30, Age-Standardized, Estimates by Country." World Health Organization. https://apps.who.int/gho/data/node.main.A900A?lang=en. Accessed May 12, 2023.

Ravn, A. M., Gregersen, N. T., Christensen, R., Rasmussen, L. G., Hels, O., Belza, A., Raben, A., Larsen, T. M., Toubro, S., and Astrup, A. "Thermic Effect of a Meal and Appetite in Adults: An Individual Participant Data Meta-Analysis of Meal-Test Trials." *Food and Nutrition Research* 57 (2013). https://doi.org/10.3402/fnr.v57i0.19676.

Bartlett, A., and Kleiner, M. "Dietary Protein and the Intestinal Microbiota: An Understudied Relationship." *iScience* 25, no. 11 (2022): 105313. https://doi.org/10.1016/j.isci.2022.105313.

Zhang, H., et al. "Meat Consumption and Risk of Incident Dementia: Cohort Study of 493,888 UK Biobank Participants." *The American Journal of Clinical Nutrition* 114, no. 1 (2021): 175–184. https://doi.org/10.1093/ajcn/nqab028.

Wan, Y., Wang, F., Yuan, J., Li, J., Jiang, D., Zhang, J., Li, H., Wang, R., Tang, J., Huang, T., Zheng, J., Sinclair, A. J., Mann, J., and Li, D. "Effects of Dietary Fat on Gut Microbiota and Faecal Metabolites, and Their Relationship with Cardiometabolic Risk Factors: A 6-Month Randomised Controlled-Feeding Trial." *Gut* 68, no. 8 (2019): 1417–1429. https://doi.org/10.1136/gutjnl-2018-317609.

Wolters, M., Ahrens, J., Romaní-Pérez, M., Watkins, C., Sanz, Y., Benítez-Páez, A., Stanton, C., and Günther, K. "Dietary Fat, the Gut Microbiota, and Metabolic Health—A Systematic Review Conducted Within the MyNewGut Project." *Clinical Nutrition* 38, no. 6 (2019): 2504–2520. https://doi.org/10.1016/j.clnu.2018.12.024.

Mattavelli, E., Catapano, A. L., and Baragetti, A. "Molecular Immune-Inflammatory Connections between Dietary Fats and Atherosclerotic Cardiovascular Disease: Which Translation into Clinics?" *Nutrients* 13, no. 11 (2021): 3768. https://doi.org/10.3390/nu13113768.

Wan, Y., Tang, J., Li, J., Li, J., Yuan, J., Wang, F., and Li, D. "Contribution of Diet to Gut Microbiota and Related Host Cardiometabolic Health: Diet-Gut Interaction in Human Health." *Gut Microbes* 11, no. 3 (2020): 603–609. https://doi.org/10.1080/19490976.2019.1697149.

Korat, A., and Victor, A. "Dairy Products and Cardiometabolic Health Outcomes." Harvard University, November 2018. https://dash.harvard.edu/handle/1/37925665.

Ristow, M., and Schmeisser, K. "Mitohormesis: Promoting Health and Lifespan by Increased Levels of Reactive Oxygen Species (ROS)." *Dose Response* 12, no. 2 (2014): 288–341. https://doi.org/10.2203/dose-response.13-035.Ristow.

Satokari, R. "High Intake of Sugar and the Balance between Pro- and Anti-Inflammatory Gut Bacteria." *Nutrients* 12, no. 5 (2020): 1348. https://doi.org/10.3390/nu12051348.

Shil, A., and Chichger, H. "Artificial Sweeteners Negatively Regulate Pathogenic Characteristics of Two Model Gut Bacteria, *E. coli* and *E. faecalis.*" *International Journal of Molecular Sciences* 22, no. 10 (2021): 5228. https://doi.org/10.3390 /ijms22105228.

Burke, M. V., and Small, D. M. "Physiological Mechanisms by which Non-Nutritive Sweeteners May Impact Body Weight and Metabolism." *Physiology & Behavior* 152, part B (2015): 381–388. https://doi.org/10.1016/j.physbeh.2015.05.036.

Jameel, F., Phang, M., Wood, L. G., and Garg, M. L. "Acute Effects of Feeding Fructose, Glucose and Sucrose on Blood Lipid Levels and Systemic Inflammation." *Lipids in Health and Disease* 13 (2014): 195. https://doi.org/10.1186/1476-511X-13-195.

Ma, X., Nan, F., Liang, H., Shu, P., Fan, X., Song, X., Hou, Y., and Zhang, D. "Excessive Intake of Sugar: An Accomplice of Inflammation." *Frontiers in Immunology* 13 (2022): 988481. https://doi.org/10.3389/fimmu.2022.988481.

Basson, A. R., Rodriguez-Palacios, A., and Cominelli, F. "Artificial Sweeteners: History and New Concepts on Inflammation." *Frontiers in Nutrition* 8 (2021): 746247. https: //doi.org/10.3389/fnut.2021.746247.

Doctrow, B. "Erythritol and Cardiovascular Events." *NIH Research Matters,* March 14, 2023. www.nih.gov/news-events/nih-research-matters/erythritol-cardiovascular-events.

Debras, C., Chazelas, E., et al. "Artificial Sweeteners and Risk of Cardiovascular Diseases: Results from the Prospective NutriNet-Santé Cohort." *PLoS Medicine* 19, no. 3 (2022): e071204. https://doi.org/10.1371/journal.pmed.1003950.

Wang, Q., et al. "Sucralose Promotes Food Intake Through NPY and a Neuronal Fasting Response." *Cell Metabolism* 24, no. 1 (2016): 75–90. http://dx.doi.org/10.1016/j .cmet.2016.06.010.

Pearlman, M., Obert, J., and Casey, L. "The Association Between Artificial Sweeteners and Obesity." *Current Gastroenterology Reports* 19, no. 12 (2017): 64. https://doi.org /10.1007/s11894-017-0602-9.

Ma, X., Nan, F., Liang, H., Shu, P., Fan, X., Song, X., Hou, Y., and Zhang, D. "Excessive Intake of Sugar: An Accomplice of Inflammation." *Frontiers in Immunology* 13 (2022): 988481. https://doi.org/10.3389/fimmu.2022.988481.

Molteni, R., Barnard, R. J., Ying, Z., Roberts, C. K., and Gómez-Pinilla, F. "A High-Fat, Refined Sugar Diet Reduces Hippocampal Brain-Derived Neurotrophic Factor, Neuronal Plasticity, and Learning." *Neuroscience* 112, no. 4 (2002): 803–814. https://doi .org/10.1016/S0306-4522(02)00123-9.

Burke, M. V., and Small, D. M. "Physiological Mechanisms by which Non-Nutritive Sweeteners May Impact Body Weight and Metabolism." *Physiology & Behavior* 152, part B (2015): 381–388. https://doi.org/10.1016/j.physbeh.2015.05.036.

Zick, S. M., Murphy, S. L., and Colacino, J. "Association of Chronic Spinal Pain with Diet Quality." *PAIN Reports* 5, no. 5 (2020): e837. https://doi.org/10.1097/PR9 .0000000000000837.

Extra-Delicious Special Section: 30 Plants in Just 5 Smoothies

Kung, B., Anderson, G. H., et al. "Effect of Milk Protein Intake and Casein-to-Whey Ratio in Breakfast Meals on Postprandial Glucose, Satiety Ratings, and Subsequent Meal Intake." *Journal of Dairy Science* 101, no. 10 (2018): 8688–8701. https://doi.org /10.3168/jds.2018-14419.

Ghazzawi, H. A., and Mustafa, S. "Effect of High-Protein Breakfast Meal on Within-Day Appetite Hormones: Peptide YY, Glucagon Like Peptide-1 in Adults." *Clinical Nutrition Experimental* 28 (2019): 111–122. https://doi.org/10.1016/j.yclnex.2019.09.002.

3. The 7-Day Challenge, and Why We Need It Now

David, L. A., Maurice, C. F., Carmody, R. N., Gootenberg, D. B., Button, J. E., Wolfe, B. E., Ling, A. V., Devlin, A. S., Varma, Y., Fischbach, M. A., Biddinger, S. B., Dutton. R. J., and Turnbaugh, P. J. "Diet Rapidly and Reproducibly Alters the Human Gut Microbiome." *Nature* 505 (2014): 559–563. https://doi.org/10.1038/nature12820.

Bourdeau-Julien, I., Castonguay-Paradis, S., Rochefort, G., et al. "The Diet Rapidly and Differentially Affects the Gut Microbiota and Host Lipid Mediators in a Healthy Population." *Microbiome* 11, no. 26 (2023). https://doi.org/10.1186/s40168-023-01469-2.

Boscaini, S., Skuse, P., Nilaweera, K. N., Cryan, J. F., and Cotter, P. D. "The 'Whey' to Good Health: Whey Protein and Its Beneficial Effect on Metabolism, Gut Microbiota and Mental Health." *Trends in Food Science & Technology* 133 (2023): 1–14. https://doi.org/10.1016/j.tifs.2022.12.009.

Sanchez-Moya, T., López-Nicolás, R. et al. "In Vitro Modulation of Gut Microbiota by Whey Protein to Preserve Intestinal Health." *Food & Function* 9 (2017). https://doi.org/10.1039/C7FO00197E.

Bartlett, A., and Kleiner, M. "Dietary Protein and the Intestinal Microbiota: An Understudied Relationship." *iScience* 25, no. 11 (2022): 105313. https://doi.org/10.1016/j.isci.2022.105313.

Wu, S., Bhat, Z. F., Gounder, R. S., Mohamed Ahmed, I. A., Al-Juhaimi, F. Y., Ding, Y., Bekhit, A. E. A. "Effect of Dietary Protein and Processing on Gut Microbiota-A Systematic Review." *Nutrients* 14, no. 3 (2022): 453. https://doi.org/10.3390/nu14030453.

4. How the Full-Body Fat Fix Will Save Your Life (Over and Over Again)

Henein, M. Y., Vancheri, S., Longo, G., and Vancheri, F. "The Role of Inflammation in Cardiovascular Disease." *International Journal of Molecular Sciences* 23, no. 21(2022): 12906. https://doi.org/10.3390/ijms232112906.

Ridker, P. M., Everett, B. M., Thuren, T., MacFadyen, J. G., Chang, W. H., Ballantyne, C., Fonseca, F., Nicolau, J., Koenig, W., Anker, S. D., et al. "Antiinflammatory Therapy with Canakinumab for Atherosclerotic Disease." *New England Journal of Medicine* 377 (2017): 1119–1131. https://doi.org/10.1056/NEJMoa1707914.

Mohammed, I., Hollenberg, M.D., Ding, H., and Triggle, C. R. "A Critical Review of the Evidence That Metformin Is a Putative Anti-Aging Drug That Enhances Healthspan and Extends Lifespan." *Frontiers in Endocrinology* (Lausanne) 12 (2021): 718942. https://doi.org/10.3389/fendo.2021.718942.

Maier, H. E., et al. "Obesity Increases the Duration of Influenza A Virus Shedding in Adults." *The Journal of Infectious Diseases* 218, no. 9 (2018): 1378–1382. https://doi.org/10.1093/infdis/jiy370.

Pugliese, G., Liccardi, A., Graziadio, C., et al. "Obesity and Infectious Diseases: Pathophysiology and Epidemiology of a Double Pandemic Condition." *International Journal of Obesity* 46 (2022): 449–465. https://doi.org/10.1038/s41366-021-01035-6.

Kay, J., Thadhani, E., Samson, L., and Engelward, B. "Inflammation-Induced DNA Damage, Mutations and Cancer." *DNA Repair* 83 (2019): 102673. https://doi.org/10.1016/j.dnarep.2019.102673.

Jackson, M. A., Jeffery, I. B., Beaumont, M., Bell, J. T., Clark, A. G., Ley, R. E., O'Toole, P. W., Spector, T. D., and Steves, C. J. "Signatures of Early Frailty in the Gut Microbiota." *Genome Medicine* 8, no. 1 (2016): 8. https://doi.org/10.1186/s13073-016-0262-7. Erratum in: *Genome Medicine* 8, no. 1 (2016): 21. Jackson, Matt [corrected to Jackson, Matthew A].

Wilmanski, T., et al. "Gut Microbiome Pattern Reflects Healthy Ageing and Predicts Survival in Humans." *Nature Metabolism* 3, no. 2 (2021): 274–286. https://doi.org/10.1038/s42255-021-00348-0.

Bredella, M. A., Torriani, M., Ghomi, R. H., Thomas, B. J., Brick, D. J., Gerweck, A. V., Rosen, C. J., Klibanski, A., Miller, K. K. "Vertebral Bone Marrow Fat is Positively Associated with Visceral Fat and Inversely Associated with IGF-1 in Obese Women." *Obesity* 19, no. 1 (2011): 49–53. https://doi.org/10.1038/oby.2010.106.

5. Listening in on the Conversation Between Your Belly and Your Brain

Radjabzadeh, D., Bosch, J. A., Uitterlinden, A. G., et al. "Gut Microbiome-Wide Association Study of Depressive Symptoms." *Nature Communications* 13 (2022): 7128. https://doi.org/10.1038/s41467-022-34502-3.

Galland, L. "The Gut Microbiome and the Brain." *Journal of Medicinal Food* 17, no. 12 (2014): 1261–1272. https://doi.org/10.1089/jmf.2014.7000.

Chinna, M. A., Forth, E., Wallace, C. J. K., and Milev, R. "Effect of Fecal Microbiota Transplant on Symptoms of Psychiatric Disorders: A Systematic Review." *BMC Psychiatry* 20, no. 1 (2020): 299. https://doi.org/10.1186/s12888-020-02654-5.

Chen, Y., Xu, J., and Chen, Y. "Regulation of Neurotransmitters by the Gut Microbiota and Effects on Cognition in Neurological Disorders." *Nutrients* 13, no. 6 (2021): 2099. https://doi.org/10.3390/nu13062099.

Messaoudi, M., Lalonde, R., Violle, N., et al. "Assessment of Psychotropic-Like Properties of a Probiotic Formulation (Lactobacillus helveticus R0052 and Bifidobacterium longum R0175) in Rats and Human Subjects." *British Journal of Nutrition* 105 (2011): 755–764. https://doi.org/10.1017/S0007114510004319.

Benton, D., Williams, C., and Brown, A. "Impact of Consuming a Milk Drink Containing a Probiotic on Mood and Cognition." *European Journal of Clinical Nutrition* 61 (2007): 355–361. https://doi.org/10.1038/sj.ejcn.1602546.

Lee, C. H., and Giuliani, F. "The Role of Inflammation in Depression and Fatigue." *Frontiers in Immunology* 10 (2019): 1696. https://doi.org/10.3389/fimmu.2019.01696.

Anderson, R. J., Freedland, K. E., Clouse, R. E., and Lustman, P. J. "The Prevalence of Comorbid Depression in Adults with Diabetes: A Meta-Analysis." *Diabetes Care* 24, no. 6 (2001): 1069–1078. https://doi.org/10.2337/diacare.24.6.1069.

Archie, E. A., and Tung, J. "Social Behavior and the Microbiome." *Current Opinion in Behavioral Sciences* 6 (2015): 28–34. https://doi.org/10.1016/j.cobeha.2015.07.008.

Ravella, S. *A Silent Fire: The Story of Inflammation, Diet, and Disease.* New York, NY: W.W. Norton, 2022.

Wong, A., Devason, A., et al. "Serotonin Reduction in Post-Acute Sequelae of Viral Infection," Cell 186, no. 21 (2023): 4475–4494, https://doi.org/10.1016/j.cell.2023.09.013.

Chandra, S., Sisodia, S. S., and Vassar, R. J. "The Gut Microbiome in Alzheimer's Disease: What We Know and What Remains to be Explored." *Molecular Neurodegeneration* 18 (2023): 9. https://doi.org/10.1186/s13024-023-00595-7.

Gonçalves, N.G., et al. "Association Between Consumption of Ultraprocessed Foods and Cognitive Decline." *JAMA Neurology* 80, no. 2 (2023): 142–150. https://doi.org/10.1001/jamaneurol.2022.4397.

Pistollato, F., et al. "Role of Gut Microbiota and Nutrients in Amyloid Formation and Pathogenesis of Alzheimer Disease." *Nutrition Reviews* 74, no. 10 (2016): 624–634. https://doi.org/10.1093/nutrit/nuw023.

Den, H., Dong, X., Chen, M., and Zou, Z. "Efficacy of Probiotics on Cognition, and Biomarkers of Inflammation and Oxidative Stress in Adults with Alzheimer's Disease or Mild Cognitive Impairment—a Meta-Analysis of Randomized Controlled Trials." *Aging* 12, no. 4 (2020): 4010–4039. https://doi.org/10.18632/aging.102810.

Xiao, S., Chan, P., Wang, T., et al. "A 36-Week Multicenter, Randomized, Double-Blind, Placebo-Controlled, Parallel-Group, Phase 3 Clinical Trial of Sodium Oligomannate for Mild-to-Moderate Alzheimer's Dementia." *Alzheimer's Research & Therapy* 13, no. 62 (2021). https://doi.org/10.1186/s13195-021-00795-7.

Li, Y., Shao, L., Mou, Y., Zhang, Y., and Ping, Y. "Sleep, Circadian Rhythm and Gut Microbiota: Alterations in Alzheimer's Disease and Their Potential Links in the Pathogenesis." *Gut Microbes* 13, no. 1 (2021): 1957407. https://doi.org/10.1080/19490976.2021.1957407.

Bode, J. C., Bode, C., Heidelbach, R., Dürr, H. K., and Martini, G. A. "Jejunal Microflora in Patients with Chronic Alcohol Abuse." *Hepato-gastroenterology* 31, no. 1 (1984): 30–34. PMID: 6698486.

Leclercq, S., Matamoros, S., Cani, P. D., et al. "Intestinal Permeability, Gut-Bacterial Dysbiosis, and Behavioral Markers of Alcohol-Dependence Severity." *Proceedings of the National Academy of Sciences of the United States of America* 111, no. 42 (2014): E4485–E4493. https://doi.org/10.1073/pnas.1415174111.

Bajaj, J. S., Gavis, E. A., Fagan, A., Wade, J. B., Thacker, L. R., Fuchs, M., et al. "A Randomized Clinical Trial of Fecal Microbiota Transplant for Alcohol Use Disorder." *Hepatology* 73, no. 5 (2021): 1688–1700. https://doi.org/10.1002/hep.31496.

Van Bogart, K., Engeland, C. G., Sliwinski, M. J., Harrington, K. D., Knight, E. L., Zhaoyang, R., Scott, S. B., and Graham-Engeland, J. E. "The Association Between Loneliness and Inflammation: Findings from an Older Adult Sample." *Frontiers in Behavioral Neuroscience* 15 (2022): 801746. https://doi.org/10.3389/fnbeh.2021.801746.

Hornstein, E. A., and Eisenberger, N. I. "Exploring the Effect of Loneliness on Fear: Implications for the Effect of COVID-19-Induced Social Disconnection on Anxiety." *Behaviour Research and Therapy* 153 (2022): 104101. https://doi.org/10.1016/j.brat.2022.104101.

Salinas, J., Beiser, A., et al. "Association of Loneliness with 10-Year Dementia Risk and Early Markers of Vulnerability for Neurocognitive Decline." *Neurology* 98, no. 13 (2022). https://doi.org/10.1212/WNL.0000000000200039.

Johnson, K. V. A. "Gut Microbiome Composition and Diversity Are Related to Human Personality Traits." *Human Microbiome Journal* 15 (2020): 100069. https://doi.org/10.1016/j.humic.2019.100069.

Sperandio, V., Torres, A. G., Jarvis, B., et al. "Bacteria-Host Communication: The Language of Hormones." *Proceedings of the National Academy of Sciences of the United States of America* 100 (2003): 8951–8956. https://doi.org/10.1073/pnas.1537100100.

Guo, G., Jia, K. R., Shi, Y., Liu, X. F., Liu, K. Y., Qi, W., Guo, Y., Zhang, W. J., Wang, T., Xiao, B., and Zou, Q. M. "Psychological Stress Enhances the Colonization of the Stomach by Helicobacter pylori in the BALB/c Mouse." *Stress* 12, no. 6 (2009): 478–485. https://doi.org/10.3109/10253890802642188.

Sun, Y., Ju, P., et al. "Alteration of Faecal Microbiota Balance Related to Long-Term Deep Meditation." *BMJ Journals: General Psychiatry* 36, no. 1 (2023). http://dx.doi.org/10.1136/gpsych-2022-100893.

Kuo, B., Bhasin, M., Jacquart, J., Scult, M. A., Slipp, L., et al. "Genomic and Clinical Effects Associated with a Relaxation Response Mind-Body Intervention in Patients with Irritable Bowel Syndrome and Inflammatory Bowel Disease." *PLOS ONE* 12, no. 2 (2017): e0172872. https://doi.org/10.1371/journal.pone.0172872.

6. The Inside Story of Your Belly

Wibowo, M. C., Yang, Z., Borry, M., et al. "Reconstruction of Ancient Microbial Genomes from the Human Gut." *Nature* 594 (2021): 234–239. https://doi.org/10.1038/s41586-021-03532-0.

Fleming-Dutra, K. E., Hersh, A. L., Shapiro, D. J., et al. "Prevalence of Inappropriate Antibiotic Prescriptions Among US Ambulatory Care Visits, 2010–2011." *JAMA* 315, no. 17 (2016): 1864–1873. https://doi.org/10.1001/jama.2016.4151.

Vallianou, N., Dalamaga, M., Stratigou, T., Karampela, I., and Tsigalou, C. "Do Antibiotics Cause Obesity Through Long-term Alterations in the Gut Microbiome? A Review of Current Evidence. *Current Obesity Reports* 10, no. 3 (2021): 244–262. https://doi.org/10.1007/s13679-021-00438-w.

Menni, C., Jackson, M. A., Pallister, T., Steves, C. J., Spector, T. D., and Valdes, A. M. "Gut Microbiome Diversity and High-Fibre Intake Are Related to Lower Long-Term Weight Gain." *International Journal of Obesity* 41, no. 7 (2017): 1099–1105. https://doi.org/10.1038/ijo.2017.66.

Hjorth, M. F., Blædel, T., and Bendtsen, L. Q., et al. "*Prevotella*-to-*Bacteroides* Ratio Predicts Body Weight and Fat Loss Success on 24-Week Diets Varying in Macronutrient Composition and Dietary Fiber: Results from a Post-Hoc Analysis." *International Journal of Obesity* 43 (2019): 149–157. https://doi.org/10.1038/s41366-018-0093-2.

Kim, M., Park, S. J., Choi, S., Chang, J., Kim, S. M., Jeong, S., Park, Y. J., Lee, G., Son, J. S., Ahn, J. C., and Park, S. M. "Association Between Antibiotics and Dementia Risk: A Retrospective Cohort Study." *Frontiers in Pharmacology* 13 (2022). https://doi.org/10.3389/fphar.2022.888333.

Noppakun, K., and Juntarawijit, C. "Association Between Pesticide Exposure and Obesity: A Cross-Sectional Study of 20,295 Farmers in Thailand." *F1000Research* 10 (2021): 445. https://doi.org/10.12688/f1000research.53261.3.

Ren, X., Kuo, Y., and Blumberg, B. "Agrochemicals and Obesity." *Molecular and Cellular Endocrinology* 515 (2020): 110926. https://doi.org/10.1016/j.mce.2020.110926.

Donaldson, D., Kiely, T., and Grube, A. "Pesticides Industry Sales and Usage: 1998–1999 Market Estimates." U.S. Environmental Protection Agency, Washington, D.C., August 2002. Report No. EPA-733-R-02-001.

Blaser, M. J. *Missing Microbes: How the Overuse of Antibiotics is Fueling Our Modern Plagues.* New York, NY: Henry Holt, 2014.

Liang, Y., Zhan, J., Liu, D., Luo, M., Han, J., Liu, X., Liu, C., Cheng, Z., Zhou, Z., and Wang, P. "Organophosphorus Pesticide Chlorpyrifos Intake Promotes Obesity and Insulin Resistance Through Impacting Gut and Gut Microbiota." *Microbiome* 7, no. 1 (2019): 19. https://doi.org/10.1186/s40168-019-0635-4.

7. Put Those Damn Vitamin Pills Down—Now!

Gahche, J., Bailey, R., Potischman, N., and Dwyer, J. "Dietary Supplement Use Was Very High among Older Adults in the United States in 2011–2014." *Journal of Nutrition* 147, no. 10 (2017): 1968–1976. https://doi.org/10.3945/jn.117.255984.

Flynn, J. "25 Fascinating Supplements Industry Statistics [2023]: Data + Trends." Zippia.com, June 27, 2023. www.zippia.com/advice/supplements-industry-statistics.

Tucker, K. "Nutrient Intake, Nutritional Status and Cognitive Function with Aging." *Annals of the New York Academy of Sciences* 1367, no. 1 (2016): 38–49. https://doi.org/10.1111/nyas.13062.

Lakhan, R., Sharma, M., Batra, K., and Beatty, F. "The Role of Vitamin E in Slowing Down Mild Cognitive Impairment: A Narrative Review." *Healthcare* 9, no. 11 (2021): 1573. https://doi.org/10.3390/healthcare9111573.

Rowland, I., Gibson, G., Heinken, A., Scott, K., Swann, J., Thiele, I., and Tuohy, K. "Gut Microbiota Functions: Metabolism of Nutrients and Other Food Components." *European Journal of Nutrition* 57, no. 1 (2018): 1–24. https://doi.org/10.1007/s00394-017-1445-8.

Ristow, M., and Schmeisser, K. "Mitohormesis: Promoting Health and Lifespan by Increased Levels of Reactive Oxygen Species (ROS)." *Dose-Response* 12, no. 2 (2014): 288–341. https://doi.org/10.2203/dose-response.13-035.Ristow.

Barzilai, N. *Age Later: Health Span, Life Span, and the New Science of Longevity.* New York, NY: St. Martin's Press, 2020.

Yeung, L., et al. "Multivitamin Supplementation Improves Memory in Older Adults: A Randomized Clinical Trial." *The American Journal of Clinical Nutrition* 118, no. 1 (2023): 273–282. https://doi.org/10.1016/j.ajcnut.2023.05.011.

"Multivitamin Improves Memory in Older Adults, Study Finds." Columbia University Irving Medical Center press release, May 24, 2023. www.cuimc.columbia.edu/news/multivitamin-improves-memory-older-adults-study-finds.

Grodstein, F., et al. "Long-Term Multivitamin Supplementation and Cognitive Function in Men: A Randomized Trial." *Annals of Internal Medicine* 159, no. 12 (2013): 806–814. https://doi.org/10.7326/0003-4819-159-12-201312170-00006.

Sinclair, D. *Lifespan: Why We Age—and Why We Don't Have To.* New York, NY: Atria Books, 2019.

Gholipour, B. "Multivitamins Are a Waste of Money, Doctors Say." *Scientific American,* December 17, 2013. www.scientificamerican.com/article/multivitamins-are-a-waste-of-money-doctors-say.

Navarro, V., et al. "Liver Injury from Herbal and Dietary Supplements." *Hepatology* 65, no. 1 (2017): 363–373. https://doi.org/10.1002/hep.28813.

"Calcium Fact Sheet for Health Professionals." National Institutes of Health, Office of Dietary Supplements. https://ods.od.nih.gov/factsheets/Calcium-HealthProfessional. Accessed April 15, 2023.

9. Muscle Out Fat

Tyrovolas, S., Panagiotakos, D., Georgousopoulou, E., Chrysohoou, C., Tousoulis, D., Haro, J. M., and Pitsavos, C. "Skeletal Muscle Mass in Relation to 10-Year Cardiovascular Disease Incidence Among Middle Aged and Older Adults: The ATTICA Study." *Journal of Epidemiology & Community Health* 74, no. 1 (2020): 26–31. https://doi.org/10.1136/jech-2019-212268.

Srikanthan, P., Horwich, T., and Tseng, C. "Relation of Muscle Mass and Fat Mass to Cardiovascular Disease Mortality." *The American Journal of Cardiology* 117, no. 8 (2016): 1355–1360. https://doi.org/10.1016/j.amjcard.2016.01.033.

Artero, E. G., Lee, D. C., Lavie, C. J., España-Romero, V., Sui, X., Church, T. S., and Blair, S. N. "Effects of Muscular Strength on Cardiovascular Risk Factors and Prognosis." *Journal of Cardiopulmonary Rehabilitation and Prevention* 32, no. 6 (2012): 351–358. https://doi.org/10.1097/HCR.0b013e3182642688.

Srikanthan, P., and Karlamangla, A. "Relative Muscle Mass Is Inversely Associated with Insulin Resistance and Prediabetes. Findings from The Third National Health and Nutrition Examination Survey." *The Journal of Clinical Endocrinology & Metabolism* 96, no. 9 (2011): 2898–2903. https://doi.org/10.1210/jc.2011-0435.

Pak, S., Park, S. Y., Shin, T. J., You, D., Jeong, I. G., Hong, J. H., Kim, C. S., and Ahn, H. "Association of Muscle Mass with Survival after Radical Prostatectomy in Patients with Prostate Cancer." *Journal of Urology* 202, no. 3 (2019): 525–532. https://doi.org/10.1097/JU.0000000000000249.

Chang, K., Hsu, T., Wu, W., Huang, K., and Han, D. "Association Between Sarcopenia and Cognitive Impairment: A Systematic Review and Meta-Analysis." *Journal of the American Medical Directors Association* 17, no. 12 (2016): 1164.e7–1164.e15. https://doi.org/10.1016/j.jamda.2016.09.013.

Boyle, P. A., Buchman, A. S., Wilson, R. S., Leurgans, S. E., and Bennett, D. A. "Association of Muscle Strength with the Risk of Alzheimer Disease and the Rate of Cognitive Decline in Community-Dwelling Older Persons." *Archives of Neurology* 66, no. 11 (2009): 1339–1344. https://doi.org/10.1001/archneurol.2009.240.

Smith, L., Firth, J., et al. "The Association of Grip Strength with Depressive Symptoms and Cortisol in Hair: A Cross-Sectional Study of Older Adults," *Scandinavian Journal of Medicine & Science in Sports* 29, no. 10 (2019): 1604–1609. https://doi.org/10.1111/sms.13497.

Li, R., Xia, J., Zhang, X., Gathirua-Mwangi, W. G., Guo, J., Li, Y., McKenzie, S., and Song, Y. "Associations of Muscle Mass and Strength with All-Cause Mortality among US Older Adults." *Medicine & Science in Sports & Exercise* 50, no. 3 (2018): 458–467. https://doi.org/10.1249/MSS.0000000000001448.

Duggal, N. A., Niemiro, G., Harridge, S. D. R., et al. "Can Physical Activity Ameliorate Immunosenescence and Thereby Reduce Age-Related Multi-Morbidity?" *Nature Reviews Immunology* 19 (2019): 563–572. https://doi.org/10.1038/s41577-019-0177-9.

Lustgarten, M. S. "The Role of the Gut Microbiome on Skeletal Muscle Mass and Physical Function: 2019 Update." *Frontiers in Physiology* 10 (2019): 1435. https://doi.org/10.3389/fphys.2019.01435.

Artero, E. G., Lee, D. C., Lavie, C. J., España-Romero, V., Sui, X., Church, T.S., and Blair, S. N. "Effects of Muscular Strength on Cardiovascular Risk Factors and

Prognosis." *Journal of Cardiopulmonary Rehabilitation and Prevention* 32, no. 6 (2012): 351–358. https://doi.org/10.1097/HCR.0b013e3182642688.

Chen, Z., Li, B., Zhan, R. Z., Rao, L., and Bursac, N. "Exercise Mimetics and JAK Inhibition Attenuate IFN-γ-induced Wasting in Engineered Human Skeletal Muscle." *Science Advances* 7, no. 4 (2021). https://doi.org/10.1126/sciadv.abd9502.

Sakuma, K., and Yamaguchi, A. "Sarcopenia and Age-Related Endocrine Function." *International Journal of Endocrinology* 2012 (2012): 127362. https://doi.org/10.1155/2012/127362.

Goodpaster, B. H., Park, S. W., Harris, T. B., et al. "The Loss of Skeletal Muscle Strength, Mass, and Quality in Older Adults: The Health, Aging and Body Composition Study." *Journals of Gerontology: Series A* 61, no. 10 (2006): 1059–1064. https://doi.org/10.1093/gerona/61.10.1059.

Cava, E., Yeat, N. C., and Mittendorfer, B. "Preserving Healthy Muscle during Weight Loss." *Advances in Nutrition* 8, no. 3 (2017): 511–519. https://doi.org/10.3945/an.116.014506.

Mangano, K. M., et al. "Dietary Protein Is Associated with Musculoskeletal Health Independently of Dietary Pattern: The Framingham Third Generation Study." *The American Journal of Clinical Nutrition* 105, no. 3 (2017): 714–722. https://doi.org/10.3945/ajcn.116.136762.

Gorissen, S., and Witard, O. "Characterising the Muscle Anabolic Potential of Dairy, Meat and Plant-Based Protein Sources in Older Adults." *Proceedings of the Nutrition Society* 77, no. 1 (2018). https://doi.org/10.1017/S002966511700194X.

Sim, M., Blekkenhorst, L., et al. "Dietary Nitrate Intake Is Positively Associated with Muscle Function in Men and Women Independent of Physical Activity Levels." *The Journal of Nutrition* 151, no. 5 (2021): 1222–1230. https://doi.org/10.1093/jn/nxaa415.

Lewis, L., et al. "Lower Dietary and Circulating Vitamin C in Middle- and Older-Aged Men and Women Are Associated with Lower Estimated Skeletal Muscle Mass." *The Journal of Nutrition* 150, no. 10 (2020): 2789–2798. https://doi.org/10.1093/jn/nxaa221.

Neville, C. E., Young, I. S., Gilchrist, S. E., McKinley, M. C., Gibson, A., Edgar, J. D., and Woodside, J. V. "Effect of Increased Fruit and Vegetable Consumption on Physical Function and Muscle Strength in Older Adults." *Age* 35 (2013): 2409–2422. https://doi.org/10.1007/s11357-013-9530-2.

Wee, A. K. "Serum Folate Predicts Muscle Strength: A Pilot Cross-Sectional Study of the Association Between Serum Vitamin Levels and Muscle Strength and Gait Measures in Patients >65 Years Old with Diabetes Mellitus in a Primary Care Setting." *Nutrition Journal* 15, no. 1 (2016): 89. https://doi.org/10.1186/s12937-016-0208-3.

Andersson, A., et al. "Fatty Acid Composition of Skeletal Muscle Reflects Dietary Fat Composition in Humans." *The American Journal of Clinical Nutrition* 76, no. 6 (2002): 1222–1229. https://doi.org/10.1093/ajcn/76.6.1222.

Smith, G. I., Julliand, S., Reeds, D. N., Sinacore, D. R., Klein, S., and Mittendorfer, B. "Fish Oil-Derived n-3 PUFA Therapy Increases Muscle Mass and Function in Healthy Older Adults." *The American Journal of Clinical Nutrition* 102, no. 1 (2015): 115–122. https://doi.org/10.3945/ajcn.114.105833.

Khor, S. C., Abdul K N., Ngah, W. Z., Yusof, Y. A., and Makpol, S. "Vitamin E in Sarcopenia: Current Evidences on Its Role in Prevention and Treatment." *Oxidative Medicine and Cellular Longevity* 2014 (2014): 914853. https://doi.org/10.1155 /2014/914853.

Dominguez, L. J., Barbagallo, M., Lauretani, F., Bandinelli, S., Bos, A., Corsi, A. M., Simonsick, E. M., and Ferrucci, L. "Magnesium and Muscle Performance in Older Persons: The InCHIANTI Study." *The American Journal of Clinical Nutrition* 84, no. 2 (2006): 419–426. https://doi.org/10.1093/ajcn/84.1.419.

Cypess, A. "Reassessing Human Adipose Tissue." *New England Journal of Medicine* 2022, no. 386 (2022): 768–779. https://doi.org/10.1056/NEJMra2032804.

Hunter, G. R., Gower, B. A., and Kane, B. L. "Age Related Shift in Visceral Fat." *International Journal of Body Composition Research* 8, no. 3 (2010): 103–108. PMC4018766.

Lobo, V., Patil, A., Phatak, A., and Chandra, N. "Free Radicals, Antioxidants and Functional Foods: Impact on Human Health." *Pharmacognosy Reviews* 4, no. 8 (2010): 118–126. https://doi.org/10.4103/0973-7847.70902.

Singal, P. K., et al. "The Role of Oxidative Stress in the Genesis of Heart Disease." *Cardiovascular Research* 40, no. 3 (1998): 426–432. https://doi.org/10.1016/S0008 -6363(98)00244-2.

Seo, D. Y., Lee, S. R., Kim, N., Ko, K. S., Rhee, B. D., and Han, J. "Age-Related Changes in Skeletal Muscle Mitochondria: The Role of Exercise." *Integrative Medicine Research* 5, no. 3 (2016): 182–186. https://doi.org/10.1016/j.imr.2016.07.003.

10. The Best Exercise Plan for Your Gut

Monda, V., Villano, I., Messina, A., Valenzano, A., Esposito, T., Moscatelli, F., Viggiano, A., Cibelli, G., Chieffi, S., Monda, M., and Messina, G. "Exercise Modifies the Gut Microbiota with Positive Health Effects." *Oxidative Medicine and Cellular Longevity* 2017 (2017): 3831972. https://doi.org/10.1155/2017/3831972.

Clarke, S. F., Murphy, E. F., O'Sullivan, O., Lucey, A. J., Humphreys, M., Hogan, A., Hayes, P., O'Reilly, M., Jeffery, I. B., Wood-Martin, R, et al. "Exercise and Associated Dietary Extremes Impact on Gut Microbial Diversity." *Gut* 63, no. 12 (2014): 1913–1920. http://dx.doi.org/10.1136/gutjnl-2013-306541.

McFadzean, R. "Exercise Can Help Modulate Human Gut Microbiota." University of Colorado, Boulder: CU Scholar. 2014. Undergraduate honors thesis 155. https://core.ac.uk /download/pdf/54845392.pdf

Grand View Research: Air Purifier Market Size, Share & Trends Analysis Report By Technology (HEPA, Activated Carbon), By Application (Commercial, Residential), By Region (APAC, Europe, MEA, North America), And Segment Forecasts, 2023–2030. Report ID: GVR-3-68038-406-2

Buffey, A., et al. "The Acute Effects of Interrupting Prolonged Sitting Time in Adults with Standing and Light-Intensity Walking on Biomarkers of Cardiometabolic Health in Adults: A Systematic Review and Meta-analysis." *Sports Medicine* 52 (2022): 1765–1787. http://dx.doi.org/10.1007/s40279-022-01649-4.

Clauss, M., Gerard, P., Mosca, A., and Leclerc, M. "Interplay Between Exercise and Gut Microbiome in the Context of Human Health and Performance." *Frontiers in Nutrition* 8, no. 10 (2021). https://doi.org/10.3389/fnut.2021.637010.

Zhao, X., Zhang, Z., et al. "Response of Gut Microbiota to Metabolite Changes Induced by Endurance Exercise." *Frontiers in Microbiology* 9, no. 20 (2018). https://doi.org/10.3389/fmicb.2018.00765.

Motiani, K. K., Collado, M. C., Eskelinen, J. J., Virtanen, K. A., Löyttyniemi, E., Salminen, S., Nuutila, P., Kalliokoski, K. K., and Hannukainen, J. C. "Exercise Training Modulates Gut Microbiota Profile and Improves Endotoxemia." *Medicine & Science in Sports & Exercise* 52, no. 1 (2020): 94–104. https://doi.org/10.1249/MSS.0000000000002112.

Bycura, D., Santos, A. C., Shiffer, A., Kyman, S., Winfree, K., Sutliffe, J., Pearson, T., Sonderegger, D., Cope, E., and Caporaso, J. G. "Impact of Different Exercise Modalities on the Human Gut Microbiome." *Sports* 9, no. 2 (2021): 14. https://doi.org/10.3390/sports9020014.

Roslund, M., Puhakka, R., et al. "Biodiversity Intervention Enhances Immune Regulation and Health-Associated Commensal Microbiota Among Daycare Children." *Science Advances* 6, no. 42 (2020). https://doi.org/10.1126/sciadv.aba2578.

McNamara, M. P., Cadney, M.D., Castro, A. A., Hillis, D. A., Kallini, K. M., Macbeth, J. C., Schmill, M. P., Schwartz, N. E., Hsiao, A., and Garland, T. "Oral Antibiotics Reduce Voluntary Exercise Behavior in Athletic Mice." *Behavioural Processes* 199 (2022): 104650. https://doi.org/10.1016/j.beproc.2022.104650.

Fayock, K., Voltz, M., Sandella, B., Close, J., Lunser, M., and Okon, J. "Antibiotic Precautions in Athletes." *Sports Health* 6, no. 4 (2014): 321–325. https://doi.org/10.1177/1941738113506553.

Cronin, O., Barton, W., Skuse, P., Penney, N. C., Garcia-Perez, I., Murphy, E. F., Woods, T., Nugent, H., Fanning, A., Melgar, S., Falvey, E. C., Holmes, E., Cotter, P. D., O'Sullivan, O., Molloy, M. G., and Shanahan, F. "A Prospective Metagenomic and Metabolomic Analysis of the Impact of Exercise and/or Whey Protein Supplementation on the Gut Microbiome of Sedentary Adults." *mSystems* 3, no. 3 (2018). https://doi.org/10.1128/mSystems.00044-18.

Cullen, J., Shahzad, S., et al. "The Effects of 6 Weeks of Resistance Training on the Gut Microbiome and Cardiometabolic Health in Young Adults with Overweight and Obesity." https://doi.org/10.1101/2023.01.27.23285016.

13. Troubleshooting the Full-Body Fat Fix

Tripathi, A. K., et al. "Molecular and Pharmacological Aspects of Piperine as a Potential Molecule for Disease Prevention and Management: Evidence from Clinical Trials." *Beni-Suef University Journal of Basic and Applied Sciences* 11, no. 1 (2022): 16 https://doi.org/10.1186/s43088-022-00196-1.

Gill, C., et al. "Watercress Supplementation in Diet Reduces Lymphocyte DNA Damage and Alters Blood Antioxidant Status in Healthy Adults." *The American Journal of Clinical Nutrition* 85, no. 2 (2007): 504–510. https://doi.org/10.1093/ajcn/85.2.504.

Es-safi, I., et al. "The Potential of Parsley Polyphenols and Their Antioxidant Capacity to Help in the Treatment of Depression and Anxiety: An In Vivo Subacute Study." *Molecules* 26, no. 7 (2021): 2009. https://doi.org/10.3390/molecules26072009.

Bouzari, A., Holstege, D., and Barrett, D. "Vitamin Retention in Eight Fruits and Vegetables: A Comparison of Refrigerated and Frozen Storage." *Journal of Agricultural and Food Chemistry* 63, no. 3 (2015): 957–962. https://doi.org/10.1021/jf5058793.

Index

About the Author

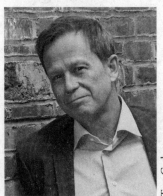

Tom Corbett

Stephen Perrine is the *New York Times* bestselling author of *The Whole Body Reset*; the cocreator, editor, and publisher of the Eat This, Not That! book series; and the cocreator of *Better Man*, a national health and wellness TV show. The former editorial creative director of *Men's Health*, as well as the former publisher of Rodale Books, he has appeared on *The View, Today, Good Morning America*, and more. He currently manages all health and wellness content for AARP Publications.